Haase®
Myotherapy

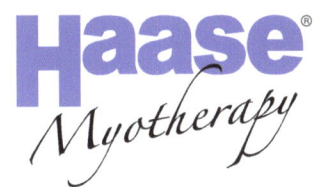

Proudly Presents...

SECRETS
of Therapeutic
BREAST MASSAGE ™

a Haase Myotherapy Course Curriculum

The publisher and author are not responsible as a matter of product liability, negligence or otherwise for any injury resulting from any material or instructions contained herein. This publication contains information relating to general principles of medical massage theory and technique which should not be construed as specific instructions for treatment of individual clients or patients.

The Secrets of Therapeutic Breast Massage™ course is typically presented live with a combination of hands-on training, lecture, and communication exercises. This course manual does not include all of the course lecture content presented in Haase Myotherapy's live continuing education classes and is not intended to be used as a stand-alone training.

Limit of Liability and Disclaimer of Warranty: While the publisher and author have used their best efforts in preparing this book, they make no representations or warranties with respect to the accuracy or completeness of the contents of this book and disclaim any implied warranties of merchantability or fitness for a particular purpose, including medical care.

Cover design, photography, and illustrations provided by Haase Seminars & Consulting
Client model: Alex Siefert
Therapist model: Sara Haase

Publisher: Burton Press International
ISBN 978-1-7351710-4-3 (Paperback)
ISBN 978-1-7351710-5-0 (eBook)

BPI

Table of Contents

Introduction

Breast massage. Those two words often evoke a variety of emotions in massage therapists and their clients alike. The public seems to have little issue seeing models exposing their scantily-clad bodies in video and print advertisements, but should a woman be seen breastfeeding her newborn child in a public place, someone would no doubt call 911 to alert the authorities to the lascivious act. And why? Because breasts are overly sexualized in American culture.

As the first Director of Marketing for the National Certification Board for Therapeutic Massage & Bodywork, I had the opportunity to visit numerous schools across the country. From Hawaii to Florida, and New York to California, I observed significant disparity among massage school licensing curriculums. Most schools would only include techniques that were within the comforts of the owner or school director OR include techniques that were within the comfort zones of the owner or school director. If they weren't comfortable with a technique? The content was removed from the syllabus leaving their students without the skills to help their clients and who could benefit from their treatments.

Never let your personal issues negatively impact your client's health. When educators avoid uncomfortable topics, they instill discomfort and fear in their students who eventually pass the uneasiness along to their clients.

For decades, a significant number of massage students, massage educators, and massage therapists have allowed their emotions, fears, and painful past experiences to shape their perspectives and opinions around the topic. The good news is, breast massage can relieve a variety of symptoms as well as help in the prevention of numerous breast issues when properly administered.

The most crucial key to providing breast massage is to ensure clear communication between the therapist and the client/patient before, during, and after the treatment. Mastering communication skills is crucial for any massage therapist if they hope to minimize misunderstandings while concurrently maximizing their client's benefit from the treatment session.

Honestly, it isn't difficult to teach Secrets of Therapeutic Breast Massage™ from a technique standpoint because the techniques themselves are not complicated. What can be complicated, however, is the dynamic between client and therapist. A significant portion of the two day training is centered around how the dynamics of a client's past experiences, values, and beliefs can affect their perceptions of the breast massage session.

During the Secrets of Therapeutic Breast Massage™ course lecture, we explain how a client perceives and remembers the breast massage session is their truth—at least to them. The problem is, their truth often does not align with the facts.

I am an expert witness in cases involving male massage therapists who have been arrested for sexual misconduct. In every case, the therapist failed to ensure clear communication with their clients and patients. So how does a therapist safely provide breast massage to the public? They do so with maturity, professionalism, and good communication skills.

It is my hope that you will be able to use the knowledge you gain from this course to positively impact the lives and health of those who experience your skilled touch.

In Health,

Robert B. Haase, LMT
Founder of Haase Myotherapy®

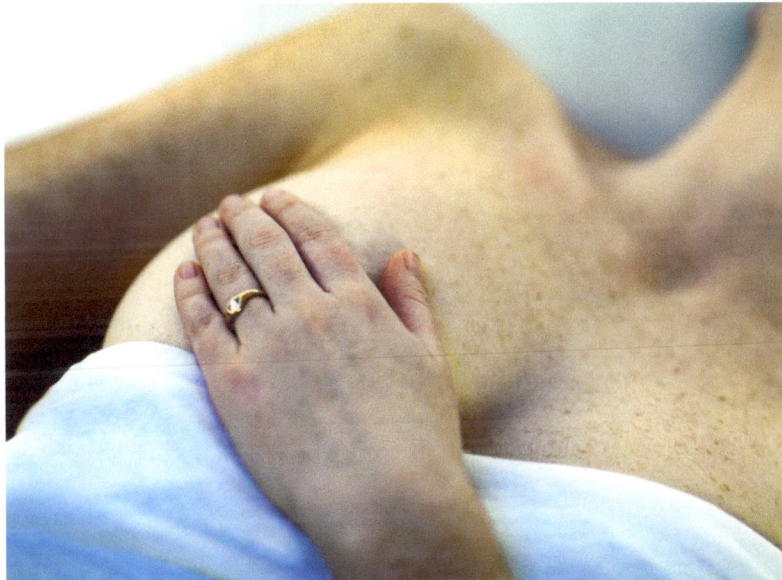

Course Overview

- Release Forms
- Communication, Ethics, Components of Client Consent
- Associated Psychology
- Anatomy, Pathology & Physiological
- Indications and Contraindications of breast massage
- Draping, therapeutic treatment techniques for a variety of breast conditions
- Expected outcomes
- Client safety related to diagnosed medical conditions

Know Your State Laws

Washington State Laws, Verbatim:

WAC 246-830-550

Standards of practice—Limitations.

- (1) It is not consistent with the standard of practice for a massage therapist to touch the following body parts on a client or patient:
- (a) Gluteal cleft distal to the coccyx, anus and rectum;
- (b) Inside the mouth unless an intraoral endorsement has been issued;
- (c) Penis;
- (d) Prostate;
- (e) Scrotum;
- (f) Vagina, to include:
- (i) Intravaginal;
- (ii) Labia (majors and minors);
- (iii) Clitoris;
- (iv) Urethra; or
- (g) Breasts, unless in accordance with WAC 246-830-555.
- (2) A massage therapist must maintain evidence of the completion of at least sixteen specialized in-person contact hours of education and training if they are performing massage in the perineal area in addition to obtaining prior written and verbal informed consent. This written consent may be included within an overall general consent to massage document, if clearly delineated and either specifically initialed or signed.
- (3) A massage therapist must not engage in sexual misconduct as described in WAC 246-16-100. Sexual misconduct will constitute grounds for disciplinary action.

WAC 246.830.005

Definitions.

- (7) "Breast massage" means the specific and deliberate manipulation of breast tissue. Massage of the surrounding chest and shoulder muscles such as massage of the intercostal, pectoral, or Axillary muscles is not considered breast massage. Breast massage is only allowed as authorized by WAC 246-830-555.

WAC 246-830-555

Breast massage.

- (1) Prior to performing breast massage, a massage therapist must:
- (a) Acquire a prior signed written consent. The written consent for breast massage may be included within an overall general consent to massage document, if clearly delineated and either specifically initialed or signed. The written consent must:
- (i) Be maintained with the client or patient's records;
- (ii) Include a statement that the client or patient may discontinue the treatment at any time for any reason;
- (iii) If the client or patient is under eighteen years of age, prior written consent must be obtained from a parent or legal guardian; and
- (iv) Include a statement that the client or patient has the option to have a witness present, and that the witness must be provided by the client or patient.
- (b) Use appropriate draping techniques as identified in WAC 246-830-560.
- (2) In addition to the requirements identified in subsection (1) of this section, a massage therapist must maintain evidence of the completion of at least sixteen hours of specialized in-person education and training in breast massage beyond the minimum competencies. Education and training in breast massage includes, but is not limited to: Breast anatomy and physiology, pathology, indications, contraindications, therapeutic treatment techniques, draping, appropriate therapist-client or patient boundaries, expected outcomes, and client or patient safety related to breast massage.
- (3) In addition to the requirements in subsections (1)

and (2), prior to performing a massage of the nipples and Areolas, a massage therapist must obtain additional documentation as follows:

- (a) A written prescription or referral from a licensed medical health care provider for this specific treatment; or

- (b) An additional prior written and verbal informed consent from the client or patient for massage of the nipple and Areolas. This written consent may be included within an overall general consent to massage document, if clearly delineated and either specifically initialed or signed.

WAC 246-830-560

Coverage and draping.

- (1) A massage therapist must:

- (a) Allow a client or patient privacy to dress or undress except as may be necessary in emergencies or custodial situations; and

- (b) Always provide the client or patient a gown or draping except as may be necessary in emergencies.

- (2) Massage therapists must use safe and functional coverage and draping practices during the practice of massage when the client or patient is disrobed. The drape(s) must be sufficient to ensure the genitals and the gluteal cleft distal to the coccyx, anus and rectum are not exposed, and the breast area is not exposed except as allowed in subsections (3) and (4) of this section. Safe and functional coverage and draping means:

- (a) The massage therapist explains, maintains and respects coverage and draping boundaries; and

- (b) Massage or movement of the body does not expose genitals or gluteal cleft distal to the coccyx, anus and rectum, or does not expose the breast area except as allowed in subsections (3) and (4) of this section.

- (3) With prior written, verbal, and signed informed consent of the client or patient, the gluteal and breast drapes may be temporarily moved in order to perform therapeutic treatment of the area. In addition, with informed and written consent, a client or patient may choose to have their upper torso undraped during the entire massage.

- (4) If variations to this coverage and draping rule occur, a massage therapist must:

- (a) Maintain evidence of education and training in specific modalities that require variations in coverage and draping;

- (b) Receive voluntary and informed consent of the client or patient prior to any variation of coverage or draping; and

- (c) Document in the client's or patient's record the rationale for any variation of coverage or draping.

- (5) Any written consent required by this section may be included within an overall general consent to massage document, if clearly delineated and either specifically initialed or signed.

WAC 246-830-565

Recordkeeping.

- (1) A massage therapist providing professional services to a client or patient must document services provided. Documentation should be appropriate to the venue, the type and complexity of those services and, when applicable, in sufficient detail to support and enable anticipated continuity of care. The documentation must include:

- (a) Client or patient name and contact information or name and contact information of a parent or guardian if a client or patient is a minor;

- (b) Age of client or patient;

- (c) Health history sufficient to ascertain if there are cautions or contraindications to safe application of massage therapy, and an update of the current health status at each session;

- (d) Date massage therapy is provided and the duration of treatment;

- (e) The types of techniques and modalities applied;

- (f) The location or areas of the body that received massage therapy;

- (g) Written consent to treat;

- (h) If breast massage is performed, an additional written consent to treat per WAC 246-830-555, and documentation of a therapeutic rationale;

- (i) If breast massage of the nipples and Areolas are involved, documentation of the prescription or referral per WAC 246-830-555 (3)(a), or an additional written consent to treat per WAC 246-830-555 (3)(b);

- (j) Documentation of any written consent or any modification in coverage and draping as required by WAC 246-830-560; and

- (k) For massage therapy where the focus is on treating a health condition, the following additional information is required:

- (i) Symptoms, for example, pain, loss of function, and muscle stiffness;

- (ii) Evaluation and findings, for example, movement, posture, palpation assessment and findings;

- (iii) Outcome measures, for example, improvement in symptoms, movement, posture, palpation, and function;

- (iv) Treatment plan for future sessions; and

- (l) If performing massage in the perineal area, an additional written and verbal informed consent to treat per WAC 246-830-550(2).

- (2) Client or patient records must be legible, permanent, and recorded within twenty-four hours of treatment. Documentation that is not recorded on the date of service must designate both the date of service and the date of the chart note entry. Corrections or additions to the client's or patient's records must be corrected by a single line drawn through the text and initialed so the original entry remains legible. In the case of computer-organized documentation, unintended entries may be identified and corrected, but must not be deleted from the record once the record is signed and completed or locked. Errors in spelling and grammar may be corrected and deleted.

- (3) Correspondence relating to any referrals by other health care providers concerning the diagnosis, evaluation, or treatment of the client or patient must be retained in the client or patient record.

- (4) Client or patient records should clearly identify the massage therapist who is the provider of services by name and signature or electronic signature and date of service.

Why Breast Massage?
- Breasts are body tissue with their own health needs

- Breast congestion; breast pain; discomfort from diagnostic and surgical procedures, lumps, and tissue changes

- Doctors, nurses and lab technicians

- Can we justify letting our inherit concerns about risk overpower our need to provide legitimate treatment?

Facts
- Breast massage in Canadian schools' curriculum

- Education is inconsistent

- Breasts are not sexual organs (NCBTMB)

- Strong association w/sexual touch/attractiveness in the USA

- There is a psycho-emotional element to breast massage

- Men need breast massage too!

- Therapeutic breast wellness/treatment massage is legal in approximately 75% of US

- Therapeutic treatment is legal in several more

- 24 states have no specific regulation for both the draping and breast massage

- 3 states require breasts to be fully draped – no further regulation (AL, DE, LA)

- 14 states have rules allowing therapist to work therapeutically and for medical treatments

Guidelines
- How to eliminate controversy….

- Always be right, know the local state law

- Mention beforehand, not day of

- Look it up

- Intonation of voice

- Compliments

- Be communicative

- Over clarify EVERYTHING!

- Draping

- Self application (teach them)

- Know your limitations

Food for Thought
- Identify your reasoning

- What do you get out of the career?

- Inadequacy/vulnerability

- Over-giving, validation, insecurities

- *Wounded Healer* Theory

- General statements

- Recognize personal weakness in professionalism

- Personal or family experiences

- Ridding our minds of past stigmas

Self-Evaluation
- Are you attracted to the client?

- Do I reveal too much non-relevant personal information?

- Do I have a need to be needed by the client?

- Do you have a need for being put on a pedestal or glorified?

- What does seeing another breast mean to you? How does it affect you?

INFORMED CLIENT CONSENT, DISCLOSURE & RELEASE

When your massage therapist provides treatment of the breast and chest area, it is important that you, the client, fully understand the nature and purpose of this treatment. In addition to discussing the massage of your breasts and breast area with your massage therapist, this written consent, disclosure and release form will act as a record of that discussion, your understanding of the treatment and your desire for your massage therapist to provide such treatment. If you have any questions, either from your discussion or while completing this form, please ask your therapist for clarification prior to signing.

☐ **I am requesting breast massage**

I,_____, after having discussed the treatment and/or treatment plan with my massage therapist, am voluntarily *requesting breast massage treatment*, for the purposes of _____

_____.

During this discussion, my therapist explained the benefits, risks and potential side effects of breast massage. I have also been informed of the areas to be treated, positioning, and how I will be draped (covered) during the massage session. I have had the opportunity to ask questions about the above information and I am aware I can ask questions at any time.

If I feel uncomfortable for any reason before or during the breast massage, I will ask the therapist to cease the treatment and continue massaging other areas, or to cease massage session. I further understand that I may modify or withdraw my consent for this treatment or the entire massage, at any time during this or any other treatment.

I understand that the nipples (areolas) of my breasts <u>will not</u> be touched at any time during the treatment. *(See additional release below if nipple/areola massage is also being requested.)*

I am comfortable having my therapist work with his or her hands directly on my uncovered breasts while performing massage.

Client Signature:_____ **Date:**_____

Witness: (<u>REQUIRED</u>) *Please check appropriate box below and **initial here**:*_____

   ☐ I am ***REQUESTING*** the option to have a witness (who I will provide) in the treatment room

   ☐ I am ***DECLINING*** the option to have a witness in the treatment room

---

CLIENT OPTIONS

Draping*: If applicable, please check appropriate box below and **initial here**:* _____

   ☐ I am ***REQUESTING*** to have ***my entire upper body exposed*** during my *entire* massage session

   ☐ I am ***REQUESTING*** to have ***my entire buttocks exposed*** while receiving related massage treatment for *purposes of:*___

_____

Nipple/Areola Massage:

In addition to my approval of receiving undraped breast massage, I am *also requesting* and clarifying my permission to receive massage treatment of my nipples and areola from my massage therapist for purposes of:_____

_____

Client Signature: _____ Date: _____

Massage therapist acknowledging receipt of this document from client after fully explaining protocols, procedures, client's rights, and client's verbal affirmation of requests noted above:

Therapist Name *(print):*_____ Therapist Signature:_____

Date of Receipt:_____

Individual Treatment SOAP Chart (female version)

Client Name: _____ Date: _____

Identify CURRENT symptomatic areas in your body by drawing the appropriate symbols on the figures below.

○ Circle areas of PAIN

✕ "X" over areas of JOINT AND MUSCLE STIFFNESS

§§ Draw wavy lines along the areas of NUMBNESS OR TINGLING

⨫ Mark RECENT SCARS, BRUISES or OPEN WOUNDS

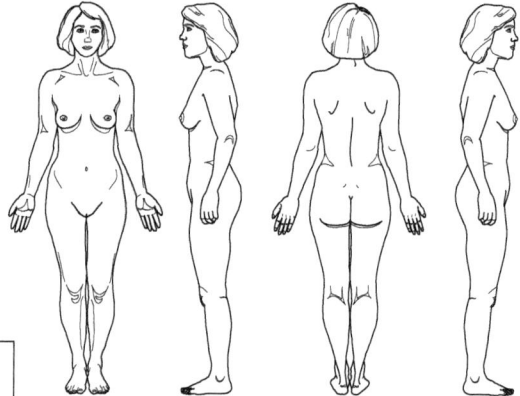

How I feel today:_____

_____

_____

_____

Confirmation of Consent: *(Client: Initial below to clarify your desire for specific treatment)*

_____ **General Consent**: *I request and authorize my massage therapist to expose, touch and provide a variety of massage techniques directly on my skin. I understand I have the right and ability to discontinue my massage treatment at at any time as well as the right to have a witness of my choosing present during my treatment.*

_____ **Breasts**: *I am requesting for my therapist to expose and massage my breasts.*

_____ **Nipple/Areola**: *I am requesting my therapist to expose and massage my nipple and/or areola*

for purposes of: _____ Rx? Y N

_____ **Upper Body Draping**: *I am requesting to have my upper body exposed during my entire massage.*

_____ **Buttocks**: *I am requesting to have my entire buttocks exposed during related massage treatment*

for purposes of:_____

Back / Posterior Shoulder:

Muscle					
Erector Spinae	L	R	B	TP	SP
Infraspinatus	L	R	B	TP	SP
Latissimus Dorsi	L	R	B	TP	SP
Psoas	L	R	B	TP	SP
Quadratus Lumborum	L	R	B	TP	SP
Rhomboids	L	R	B	TP	SP
Serratus Anterior	L	R	B	TP	SP
Subscapularis	L	R	B	TP	SP
Supraspinatus	L	R	B	TP	SP
Teres Minor / Minor	L	R	B	TP	SP
Trapezius, Upper	L	R	B	TP	SP
Trapezius, Lower	L	R	B	TP	SP
Triceps	L	R	B	TP	SP

Neck / Head:

Muscle					
Levator Scapulae	L	R	B	TP	SP
Masseter	L	R	B	TP	SP
Scalenes (Ant-Med-Post)	L	R	B	TP	SP
Splenius Capitis	L	R	B	TP	SP
Splenius Cervicis	L	R	B	TP	SP
Sternocleidomastoid	L	R	B	TP	SP
Suboccipitals	L	R	B	TP	SP
Temporalis	L	R	B	TP	SP

Legend:	B = Bilateral
L = Left	TP = Trigger Point
R = Right	SP = Spasm

Leg:

Muscle					
Adductors (upper - lower)	L	R	B	TP	SP
Biceps Femoris	L	R	B	TP	SP
Gastrocnemius	L	R	B	TP	SP
Peroneus Longus/Brevis	L	R	B	TP	SP
Quadriceps Femoris Group	L	R	B	TP	SP
Sartorius	L	R	B	TP	SP
Soleus	L	R	B	TP	SP
Tensor Fascia Latae	L	R	B	TP	SP
Tibialis Anterior	L	R	B	TP	SP

Arm:

Muscle					
Biceps Brachii	L	R	B	TP	SP
Deltoid	L	R	B	TP	SP
Extensor Group	L	R	B	TP	SP
Flexor Group	L	R	B	TP	SP
Triceps Brachii	L	R	B	TP	SP

Hip:

Muscle					
Gluteus Maximus	L	R	B	TP	SP
Gluteus Med/Min.	L	R	B	TP	SP
Illiacus	L	R	B	TP	SP
Piriformis	L	R	B	TP	SP

Chest:

Muscle					
Intercostals	L	R	B	TP	SP
Pectoralis Major	L	R	B	TP	SP
Breast*				*See Treatment Rationale	

Treatment Codes for Today:

units	97124	Massage	15min
_____ units	97124	Massage	15min
_____ units	97112	NMR	15min
_____ units	97140	Manual Tx	15min

Additional Codes _____

Co-Pay Received

$

Therapist Initials:

Additional Subjective Notes

Objective:

Treatment Rationale:

Assessment:

Plan:

Communications & Ethics

How do we communicate?

- Verbal
  - ▶ Words
  - ▶ Tone of Voice
- Facial Expressions
- Physical Gestures
- Physical Posture
- Touch

In the workplace...

- 50% of work time is spent listening…
- Immediately following a conversation, we retain HALF of what we hear…
- After 48-hours we only remember 25%
- 60% of all management problems are related to poor listening
- We interpret 70-90% of what we hear

> **Poor communication is the number one reason most massage therapists get into legal trouble.**

The best time to communicate?

- When making the appointment [Expectations]
- When the client arrives for their massage [Clear instructions]
- During your massage intake conversation [Re-clarify Expectations]
- During the massage [Clarify what you are working on and purpose, feedback on pressure, etc.]
- After the massage [Followup]
- **Note**: Never provide breast massage on the same day you bring up the topic to your patient/client, giving them time to process and consider.

Role play scenarios

- Introduce the subject to a client not currently seeking therapeutic breast massage
- Give a pamphlet with breast-massage-based content
- Verbally explain its medical benefits and application process
- Express the idea of breast massage passively through conversation

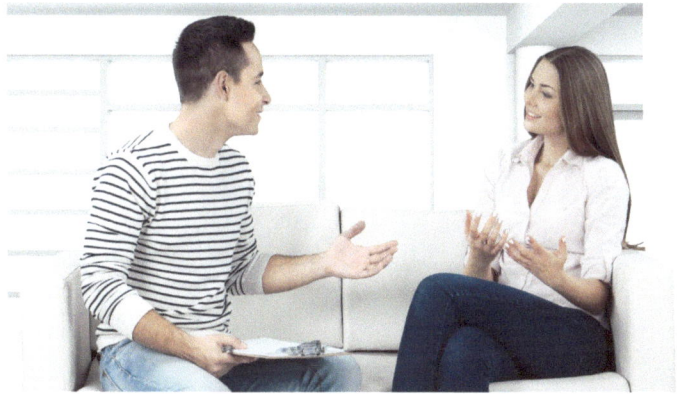

- How to approach same day massage treatment:
  - ▶ Make sure it is deemed medically necessary
  - ▶ Have consent form readily available, explain verbally, have them sign it prior, at check-in, or table side
  - ▶ Explain that the treatment can stop at any given time per their request

Gender Dynamics

- Gender issues
- Understanding client's mindset
- What experiences are they bringing into the session?
- How will a female client react to offer of breast massage? With fear? Excitement?
- Use extra caution
- Actions of "stray" therapists affecting your profession
- Referrals

Notes:

Anatomy of the Breast

Components of Client Consent

- Body language/posture/facial expression
- Clients who readily give consent
- Clients who want to be the "director"
- Different signatures, same document
- Verbal consent renewal
- Complete understanding for what and why
- Client goals are stated and wishes are in alignment with treatment
- Clarity on their rights to interject, suggest modifications
- Explain draping positioning, possible discomforts, duration of treatment and modalities used
- Client says "yes" to plan

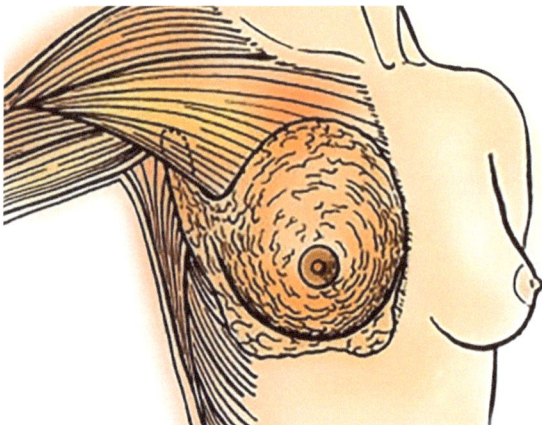

Breast Tissue Location

- Breast tissue extends beyond the breast contour above, below, and into the Axilla.

Breast Quadrants

- UIQ: Upper Inner Quadrant
- UOQ: Upper Outer Quadrant
- LIQ: Lower Inner Quadrant
- LOQ: Lower Outer Quadrant

Chest Abnormalities

- Pectus Carinatum: Anteriorly displaced Sternum
- Barrel chest: Increased anterior posterior diameter
- Pectus Excavatum (aka Pectus Recurvatum, Funnel Chest, and Cobbler's Chest)
- Depressed lower Sternum
- Thoracic Kyphoscoliosis: Raised shoulder and scapula, thoracic convexity, flared interspaces

Breast Irregularities

- Variations:
  - ► Accessory Nipple
  - ► Polymastia
  - ► Polythelia
- *Ominous Signs* suggest the possibility of a dangerous cause. This term is universally recognized to denote serious origin for signs and symptoms that are not diagnostic but warrant further investigation. Examples include:
  - ► Nipple Discharge
  - ► Nipple Retraction (aka inverted nipple or, Invaginated Nipple)
  - ► Lumps: growth that develops within the breast
  - ► Changes in Breast Contour
  - ► Changes in Skin Color and Texture
  - ► Changed Prominence of Veins

Keywords

- **Mammary** – breast or tissue of the breast
- **Mastalgia** – pain experienced in breast /cyclical mastaliga

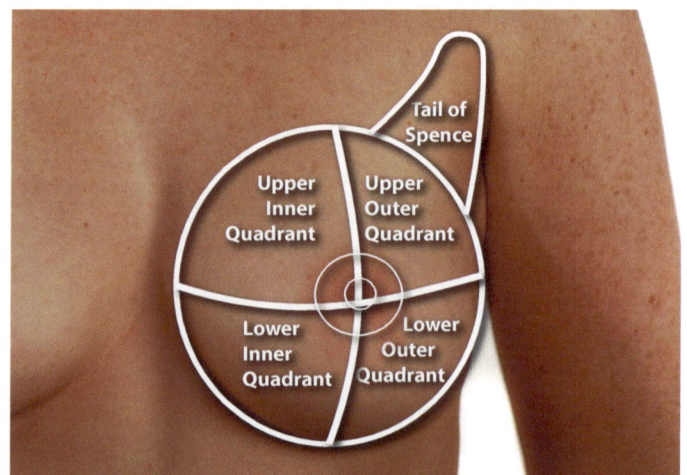

- **Mastectomy** – full or partial removal of breast
- **Radical Mastectomy** – removal of breast, Pectoralis muscles, and Axillary lymph nodes
- **Involution** – breasts recede from state of readiness for lactation; return to pre-pregnancy state
- **Parenchyma** – functional tissue (glandular structure of lobes)
- **Lactation** –period when woman's breasts are producing milk and breastfeeding

Pathologies

ANDI
(Aberrations of Normal Development and Involution)

Legend:
🟩 Massage is indicated
🟨 Massage with caution
🟧 Massage is contraindicated

Benign Breast Conditions/Disorders – NOT disease, minimal to no added risk of malignancy/cancer

- 🟩 ► **Fibrosis** –excessive connective tissue build up.
- 🟨 ► **Cyst**- Fluid filled sacs –microcyst-cyst-macrocyst (Never manipulate cysts in an effort to express the contents.)
- 🟨 ► **Oil cyst** – Post surgery or radiation can cause at necrosis, Instead of dead tissue turning into scar tissue, the body envelopes with calcium forming an oil cyst. *Massaging necrotic tissue is contraindicated. Avoid pressing on cysts directly.*
- 🟩 ► **Fibrocystic breast conditions/Changes/Diffuse Cystic Mastopathy of Unspecified Breast (ICD10)** – presents in the duct or lobe of the breast with or without fibrosis. Presents most commonly in the left UOQ.

🟩 Fibroadenosis
- Excessive connective and glandular tissue growth
- Painful nodularity or Epithelial Hyperplasia
- Generally found in UOQ
- Generally presents in ages 20-45
- Massage indicated if lumps are confirmed benign

🟩 Fibroadenomas
- Benign tumors made up of connective and glandular tissue
- Aggregate Adenosis, Tumoral Adenosis, or Adenosis tumor
- Often found in UOQ of women with fibrocystic breast conditions
- Generally presents in ages 21-69

🟩 Sclerosing Adenosis
- A special type of adenosis in which the enlarged lobules are distorted by scar-like fibrous tissue, increased acini production
- Invades nerves and blood vessels
- Generally presents in ages 35-72

🟧 Lactational Mastitis
- Inflammation of breast tissue by bacterial infection from breast feeding or blockage of a milk duct
- TX: cold compresses / 10 day antibiotics

🟧 Non-Lactational Mastitis Types
- Foreign Body
- Ganulomatous
- Idiopathic Granulomatious
- Paracitic
- Fungal
- Periductal

Notes

Duct Ectasia

- Chronic inflammation of the duct, milk duct dilates, duct walls thicken, and fills with fluid
- Also known as Mammary Duct Ectasia, Ectasia of the breast, Plasma Cell Mastitis
- TX: Warm compresses / Antibiotics, surgery or no-treatment
- Generally presents in menopausal/post-menopausal women

Intraductal Papilloma & Papillomatosis

- Benign breast lesion that occurs within lactiferous ducts, wart like in shape
- Solitary papilloma or intraductal papilloma
- Papillomatosis – very small areas of cell growth within the ducts, but they are not as distinct solitary papillomas
- TX: Surgical Removal
- Generally presents in ages 35-65
- Hot, moist heat with massage unless cancerous
- Fibrocystic breast condition
- Myalgia/cyclical myalgia
- Mastitis prevention
- Lymphedema/lipedema/congestion
- Breast trauma/scare tissue
- Drainage issues
- Assistance in monitoring
- Help with touch aversion issues

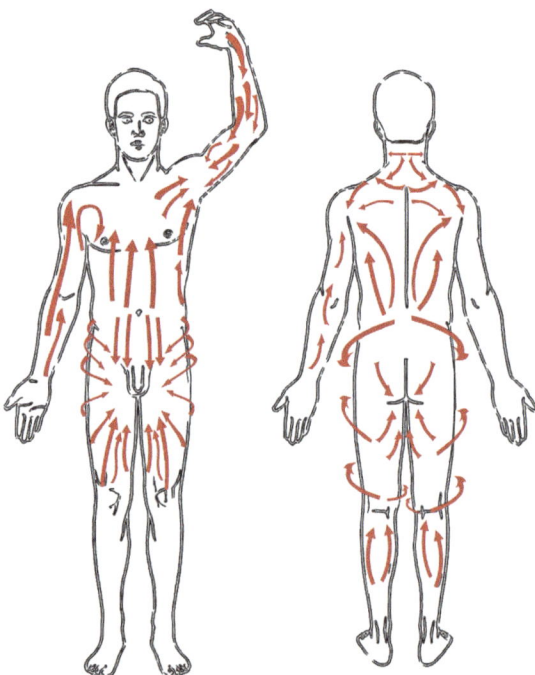

- Education in self breast massage
- Post operative
- Thoracic Outlet Syndrome
- Postpartum

Contraindications for Massage

- Mastitis/lactational mastitis
- Active infections
- Direct work on undiagnosed lumps
- Client has lateral breast and subscapular pain with sub-pecular implant (possible Serratus Anterior rupture)
- Therapist can not be professionally neutral
- Good communication does not exist
- Abscess
- Distorted contour without diagnosis
- Client refuses
- Unable to receive written consent

Lymph Flow

Lymph flows in only one direction within its own system
- The direction is upward and toward the neck
- 75% of breast lymph goes to the system of nodes in the Axilla
- 25% of the breast lymph escapes via the internal mammary chain along the Sternum
- Toxins in lymph nodes are destroyed by lymphocytes
- Right and Left
- Pressure Theory
- Damaged tissues & rerouting
- Lack of blood supply and lymphatic movement from Thoracic Outlet Syndrome (T.O.S.) increases ones risk of breast cancer.

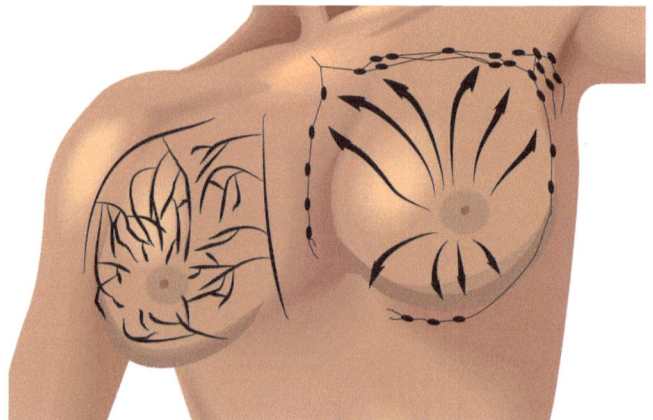

How Common is Cancer?

- About 1,685,000 new cases in 2016, 1,688,780* cases estimated in 2017
- Breast Cancer is #1 for women
  - ▶ 15% of new cancer cases
  - ▶ 89.7% 5-year survival rate
  - ▶ 6.8% of all cancer deaths
- Prostate Cancer is #1 for men
  - ▶ 9.6% of new cancer cases
  - ▶ 98.6% 5-year survival rate
  - ▶ 4.4% of all cancer deaths
- MALE Breast Cancer Estimates for 2017
  - ▶ 100 times less common for men vs women
  - ▶ Lifetime risk for men is 1 in 1,000
  - ▶ 2,470 new cases of breast cancer will be diagnosed
  - ▶ 460 men will die from breast cancer (18%)
- Techniques tailored to frailty of tissues, including s, skin and bone
- Part of a medical health care team
- Adaptive / ever-changing treatment plan
- Environment is unusual and hostile
- Profound impact of massage on patients
- Expect the unexpected

Developing a Treatment Plan

- Assess the patient
- Outline treatment plan

- Provide treatment
- Document your intervention
- Develop future plans

Assess the Patient

- Talk to nurse or doctor first
- Medical history
- Muscles, bones, body parts affected
- Specific test results and conditions
- Massage history?
- Don't play doctor

Outline Treatment Plan

- Now that you have all of the information:
  - ▶ Modality
  - ▶ Frequency / duration
  - ▶ Touch
  - ▶ Positioning
  - ▶ Privacy

Be Aware of Apparatus

- Inserted in Superior Vena Cava:
  - ▶ Mediports
  - ▶ Groshong catheter
- Shunts
- Don't react—*prepare yourself*

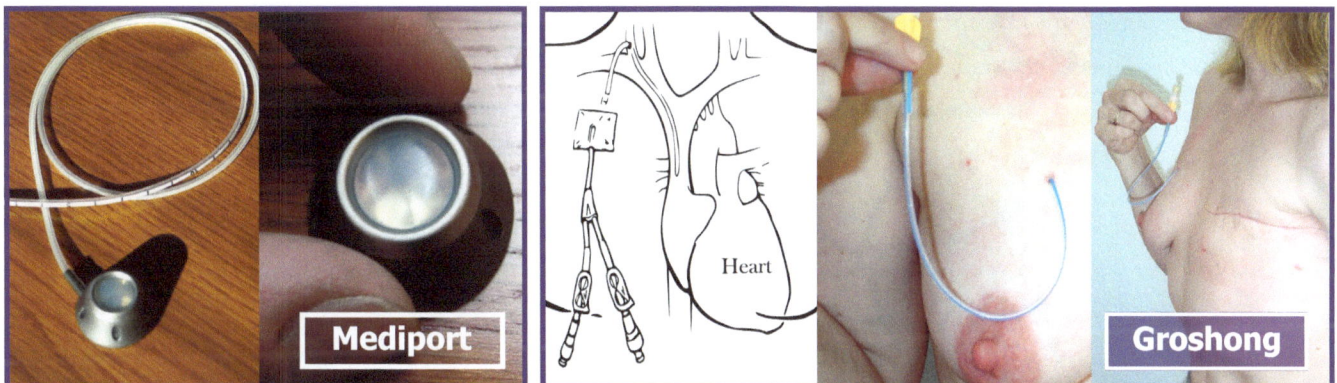

Mediport

Heart

Groshong

Massaging Cancer Patients

- Low platelet count (<50K) = bruising – do not "massage"
- Don't massage directly on/over a tumor
- Avoid matastatic sites (e.g.:Axillary)
- Don't treat if you are sick
- Wear mask / gloves if needed
- Be aware that clients will miss appointments

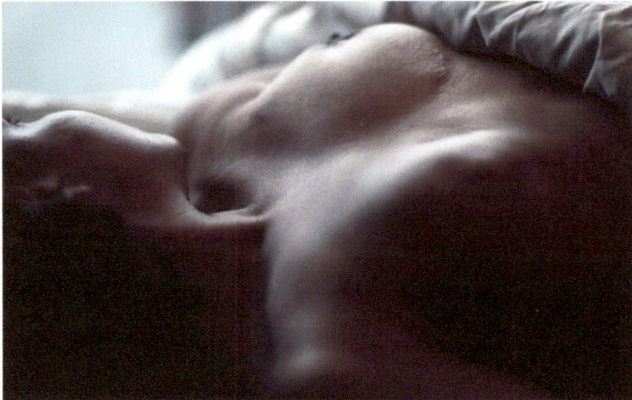

- Avoid deep tissue (even if requested)
  - ► Pain medications block normal feedback
  - ► Tissues fragile, including bones that break
  - ► Chemotherapy taxes the body of energy; deep tissue adds to that overload
- Avoid biopsy sites for a week or so
  - ► Even more time for bone marrow aspirations
- No work in surgery sites for 4-6 weeks
- Bones weaken from treatment
- Bones REALLY weaken if cancer is in them
- Inquire about blood clots
- Avoid "tattoo" / radiation sites
  - ► No creams or oils
- Be prepared with adequate bolsters
- Be prepared with moisture barriers
  - ► Caution around colostomy bags
- Pulmonary Embolism is contraindicated
- Bowel obstructions: stay clear!
- Deep Leg Thrombosis: no legs / feet
- Stay clear of weeping lesions
- Do not "dabble" in lymphatic work unless you are trained in this area
- DO NOT suggest medication/dietary changes
- Do not recommend herbs
  - ► Research shows many can interfere with liver function
- Realize that bone degradation lasts years
- Lymph vessels DO NOT regenerate
- Elevate edema when bolstering
- Be aware of wide mood swings
- Be clear before treatment starts as to how long the massage / treatment will last
- Emotions
- Fortify your tender heart
- Self-Care
- When cancer wins

Tumor Types

- Lipoma
- Hamartoma
- Hemangioma
- Hematoma
- Adenomyoepithelioma
- Neurofibroma
- Melanoma
- Phyllodes

Phyllodes Tumors - Cystosarcoma Phyllodes - Phyllodes Cystosarcoma

- Masses arise from connective tissues surrounding the ducts of the breast
- Benign/malignant potential
- Cancerous Type & TX
- Li-Fraumeni Syndrome
- Generally presents in age 50-60

Cancer Types within the Breast

- Ductal Carcinoma In Situ – Pre-invasive cancer of ductal lining
- Invasive Ductal Carcinoma – Invasive Cancer that has spread outside of the ductal lining
- Subtypes: Tubular, Mucinous, Inflammatory, Medullary
- TX: surgery, hormone therapy, radiation and chemo
- LCIS – Lobular Carcinoma In Situ – NOT cancer
- Invasive Lobular Carcinoma – Invasive cancer of the

lobular unit

- Metaplastic Cancer – The three most common types of receptors known to fuel most breast cancer growth (Estrogen, Progesterone, and the HER-2/neu gene) are not present in the cancer tumor.

Other Cancer Types

- Paget's Disease: 95% of the time it is when DCIS spreads to the Areola or nipple
- Angiosarcoma: A rare cancer that starts in the cells that line blood/lymph vessels
- Anaplastic Large Lymphoma: Affects cells in the immune system and can be found around the breast implant

Accellular Dermal Collagen Matrix Mastopexy

- An allografted donation of the dermis and epidermis skin tissue from a cadaver or animal (e.g.: pig)
- Breast lift

Breast Augmentation:

Implants & Ex-Plants
History of augmentation
- Incision Types for Augmentation
- Trans-Axillary
  - ► Peri-Areolar
  - ► Inframammary crease
  - ► Transumbilical (TUBA)
- Implant Types
  - ► Saline
  - ► Silicone Gel
  - ► Fluid/gelatenous
  - ► Cohesive silicone ("Gummy Bear Implant")
- Implant Placements
  - ► Subglandular
  - ► Subpectoral
  - ► Submuscular
- Incision Types for Augmentation
  - ► Trans-Axillary
  - ► Peri-Areolar
  - ► Infra-mammary
  - ► Transumbilical

Anomalies of Breast Implantation

- Breast implant migration – implant moves up, down or sideways in its pocket
- Filler material migration - filler material which has leaked outside of the outer shell and spread throughout the surrounding organic tissue
- Symmastia: Confluence of breast tissue across the midline anterior to the Sternum
- Capsular Contracture: A scar (or capsule) formation around implant

Notes:

Capsular Contracture & Massage

- What is Capsular Contracture?
  - ► The body reacting to a foreign body
  - ► Similar to a cyst or a pearl
  - ► Soften post-operatively
- Expedites "dropping and fluffing"
- Reduces swelling and expedites the healing process
- Prevention and TX

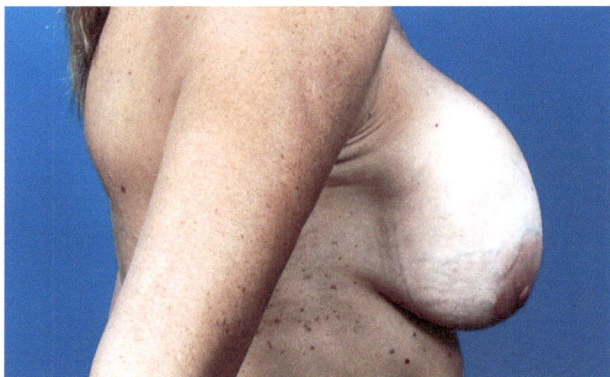

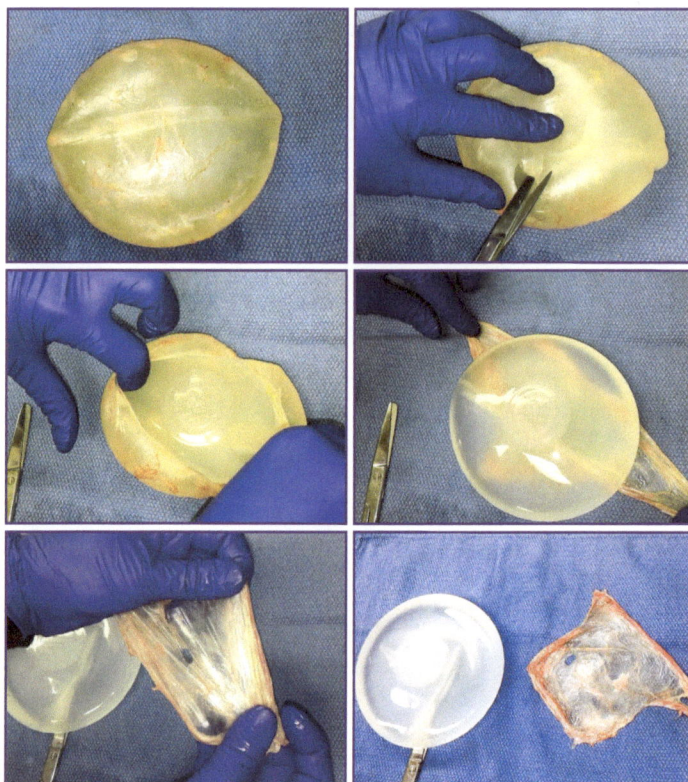

Scar Tissue and Burns

- Types: radiation, electrical, chemical, fire and liquid
- 1st degree burns – epidermis only
- 2nd degree burns - inflammatory phase, proliferate, maturation
- 3rd degree burns – skin grafting, debridement, surgeries and procedures

Scar Types

- Contracture
- Keloid
- Hypertrophic
- Dimple scar
- Varied scar lines post-mastectomy

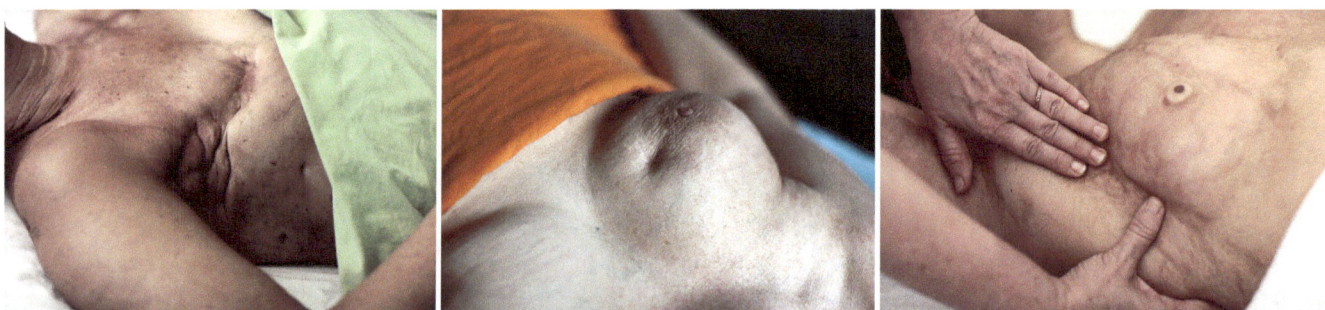

Notes:

Section Two: Technique

Haase Myotherapy's Essential Breast Massage Sequence

Purpose: Stimulate lymph flow and drainage, decrease inflammation and scar tissue formation post operatively.

Related Pathologies: Lymphedema, fibrocystic breast condition, cancer related treatment.

Indications: Myalgia, inflammation, nodularity, restriction in tissues due to trauma, client requests for general breast health.

Endangerments: Potential damage to lymph nodes, blood vessels, glandular structure, thin skin and muscles due to cancer treatments.

Expected Outcomes: Increase lymph flow, drainage, decrease in fibrocystic breast conditions (goes away completely), decrease myalgia, increase strength of stromal tissues ("perky"breast tissue), expedite healing process.

Stimulate lymph flow in the upper anterior thoracic and breast areas: Stand adjacent to your client, facing towards their head, place one hand on the Sternum with fingers held together firmly.

Tap rhythmically with your fingers against the back of your hand, transferring the percussive movement into your client's Sternum, stimulating the lymph flow.

Gently place overlapped hands on top of Sternum with "full palmar contact", overlap your hands, placing one hand directly over the other.

Gently press downward, slowly, pressing and releasing at a rate of about one compression every second, creating a smooth pumping action.

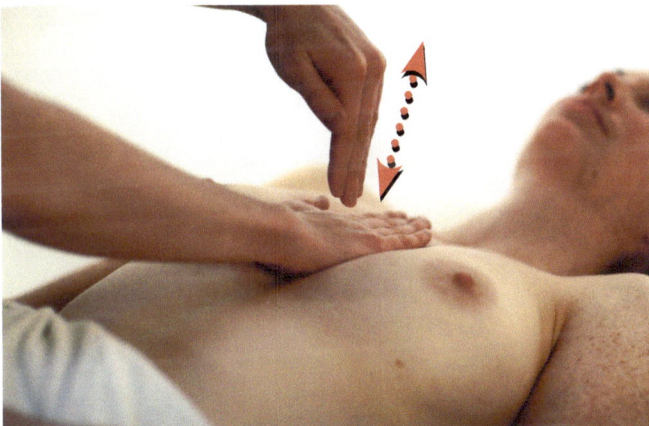

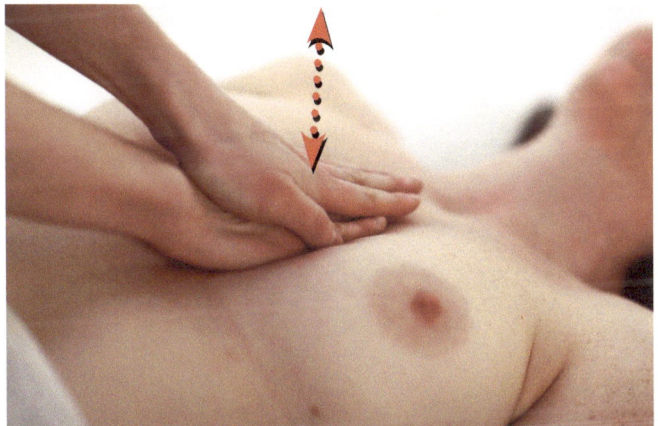

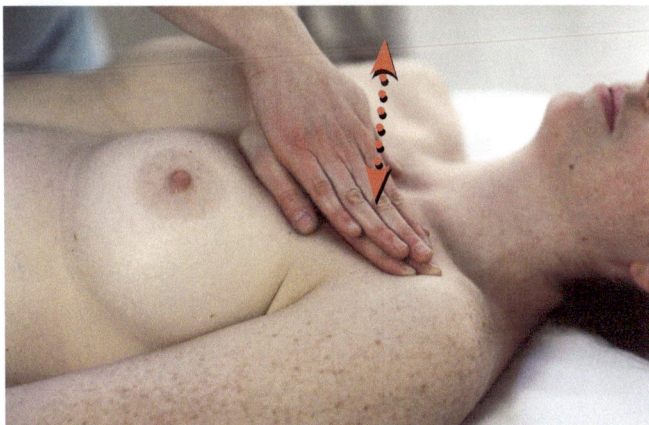

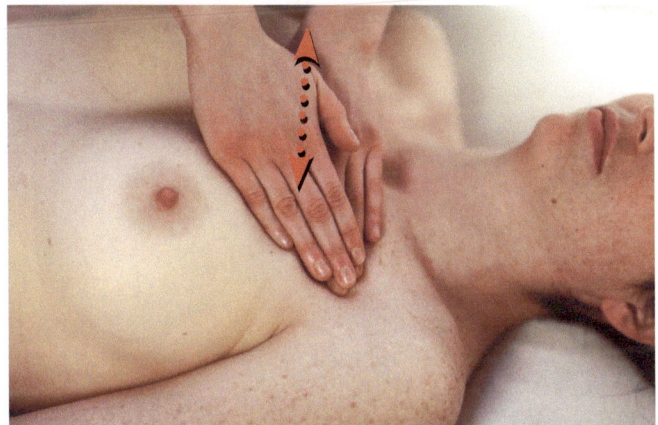

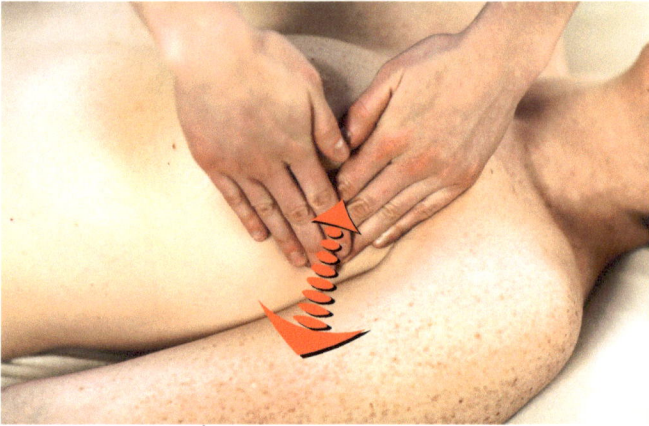

Continue with the same pumping compressions as you work around the breast and Pectoralis Major, working from the opposite side of which you are standing. Work in a direction moving up the Sternum, then up and lateral over the upper chest being sure to work up to and just under the clavicle.

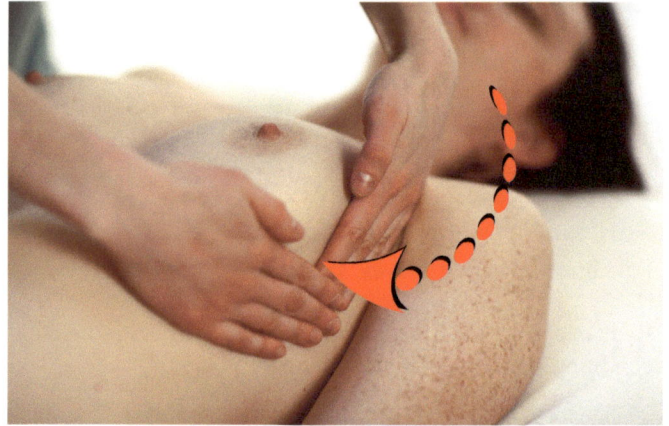

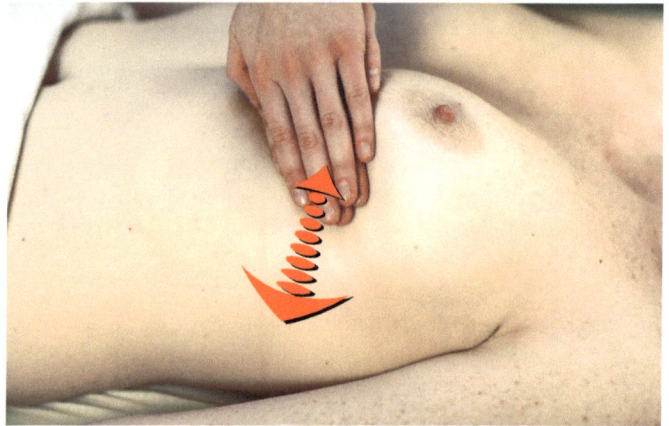

Using one hand to stabilize the breast, use two fingers on your other hand to gently squeegee the superficial tissues of the breast, gliding directly away from the nipple. Work all the way around the breast.

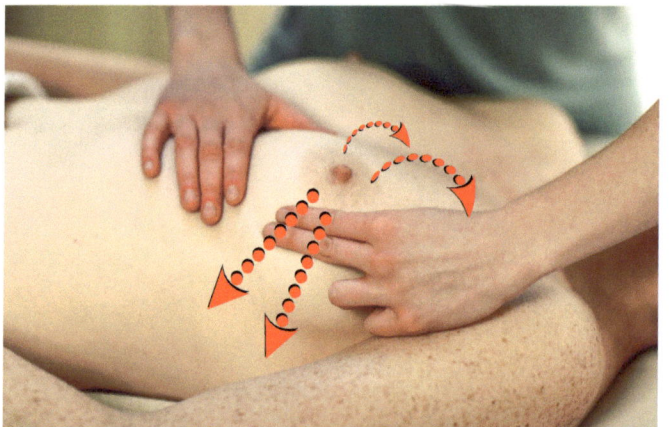

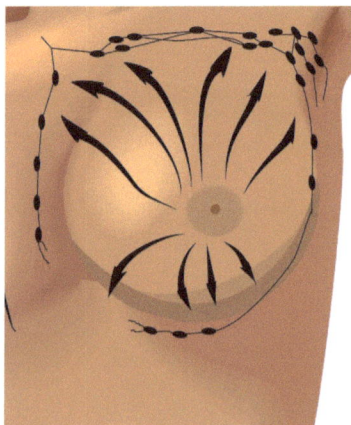

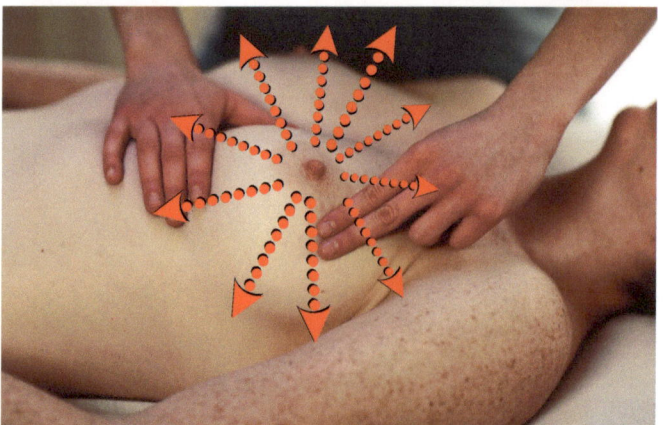

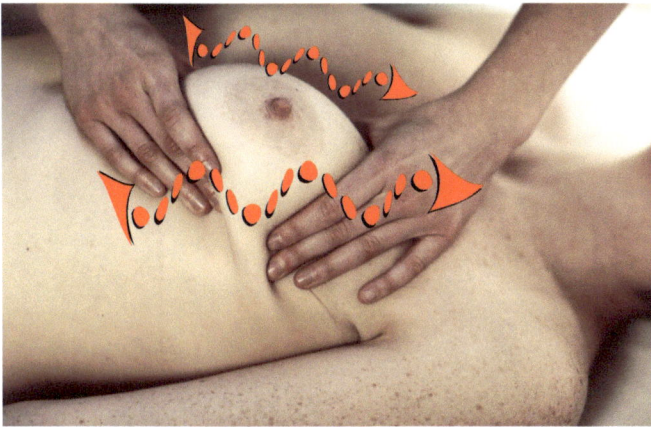

With both hands, begin massaging the entire breast with petrissage strokes, being sure to gently mobilize the tissue.

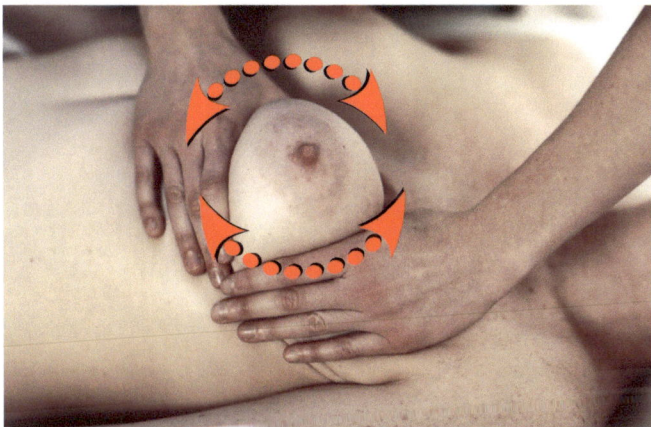

In an effort to benefit the Cooper's Ligaments of the breast, use both of your hands and twist the breast into gentle traction. Twist both clockwise and counterclockwise in alternate directions, holding each twist for 1-2 seconds before redirecting the twist in the other direction.

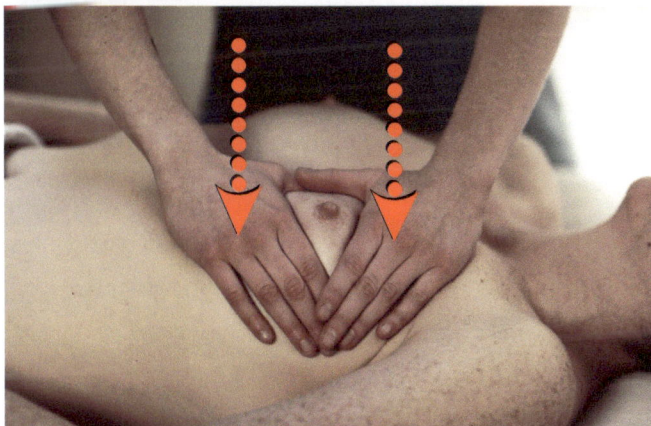

With both hands, use compressions, each lasting 1-2 seconds, pressing downward into your client's chest until the breast appears nearly flat.

Depending on your preference, you can either press with your hands encircling the Areola*, or with your hands completely covering the Areola. The preferred method is to include the Areola with each compression.

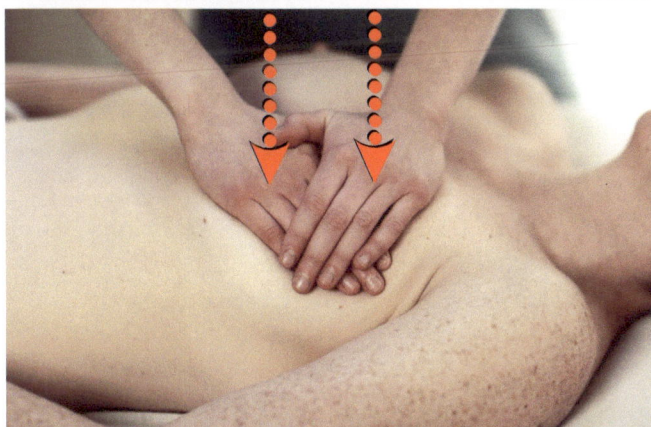

*If your state's massage laws specifically prohibit contact with the Areola and you prefer to include it in the compression, you can place the client's hand from the opposite side of the breast to be compressed over their breast. You would then press downward with the client's hand between the breast and your own hands.

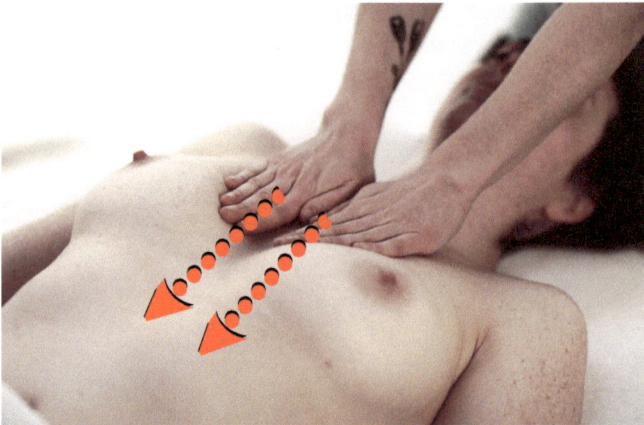

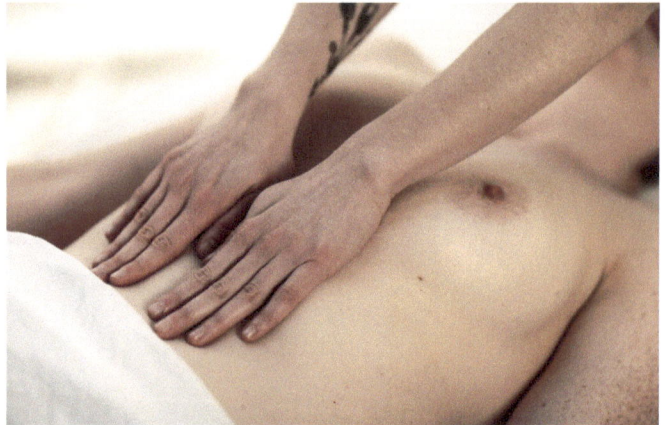

You will now finish the sequence with a traditional Hawaiian Lomi-Lomi smoothing effleurage stroke from the head of the table. Begin with your flat hands pressing down on the upper chest, gliding down the Sternum, down and over the lower abdomen.

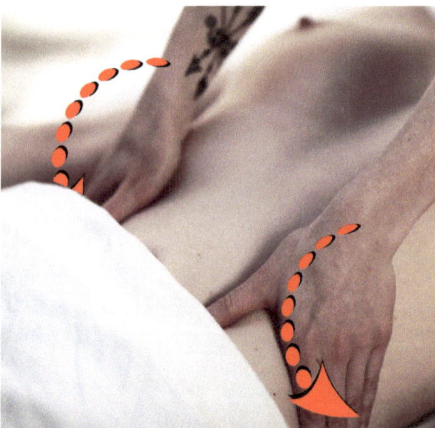

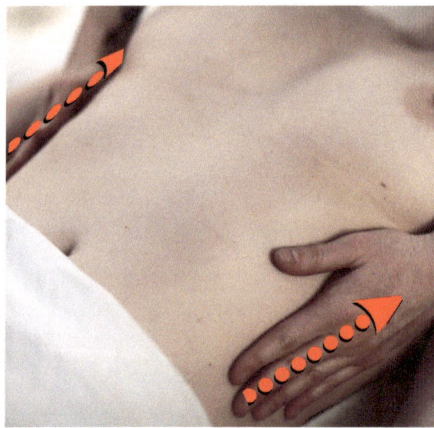

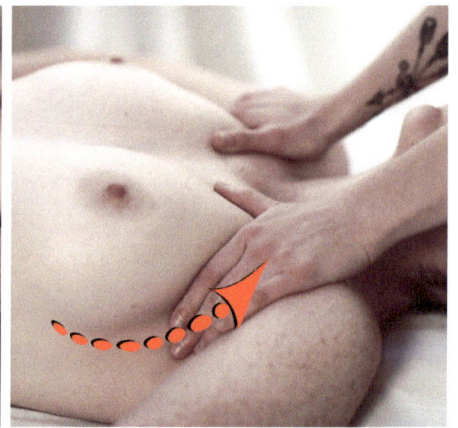

With hands mirroring each other on both sides of the anterior torso, glide laterally over External Obliques and back up along Serratus Anterior.

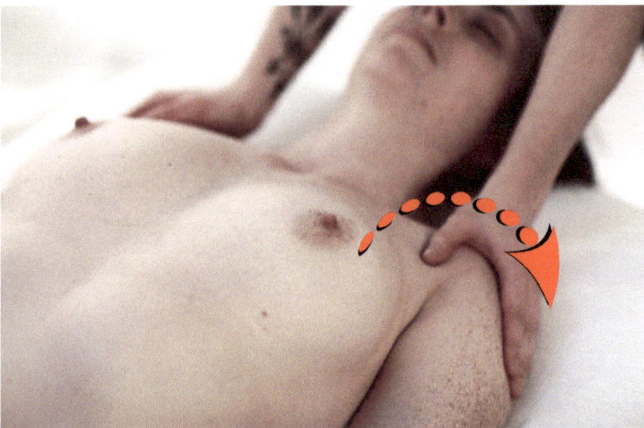

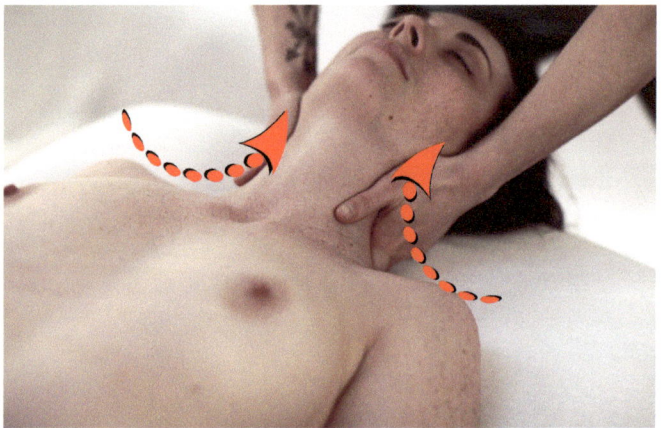

Continue the stroke along the lateral breasts, gathering together at the Sternum, just below the Menubrial Notch, and then over the Deltoids, finishing along the lateral neck with a gentle squeeze.

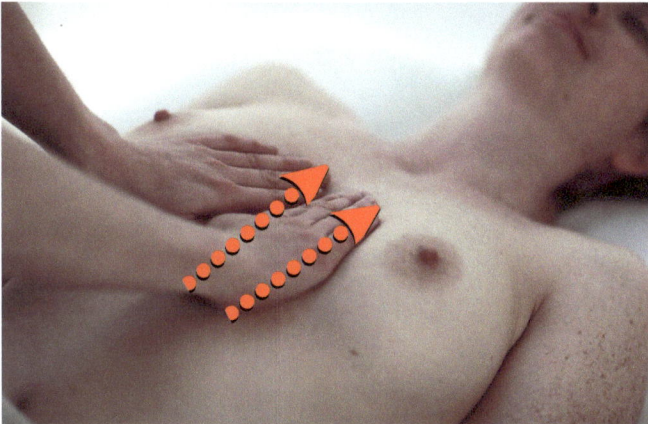

Similarly, you will repeat the previous Hawaiian Lomi-Lomi effleurage stroke from the side of the table, as you stand with your backside towards the client's feet.

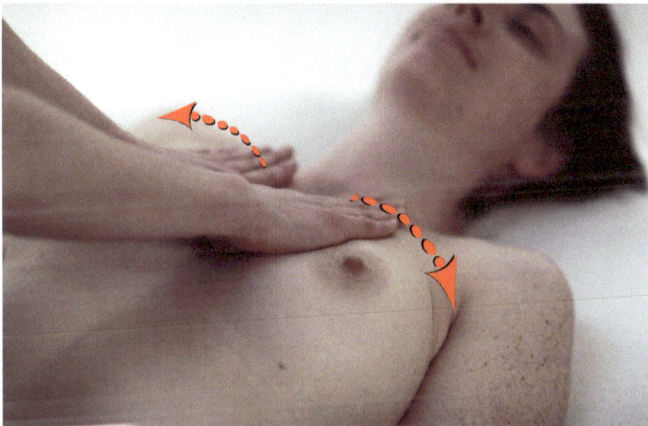

With your flat hands, side by side, begin at the center of the Sternum, gliding superiorly, up and then laterally over and around the breasts.

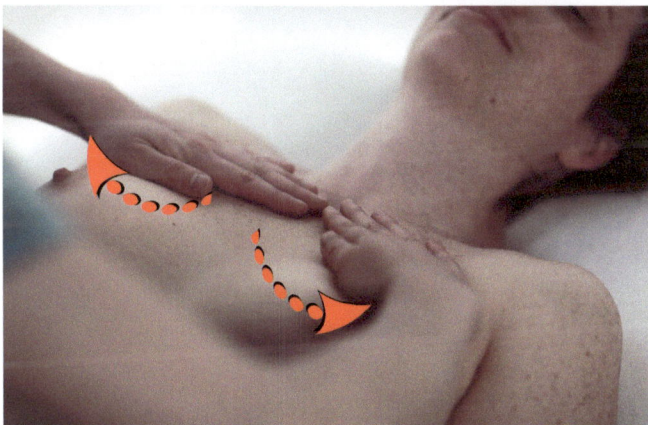

The stroke finishes as your hands come together, gathering together at the lower ribcage.

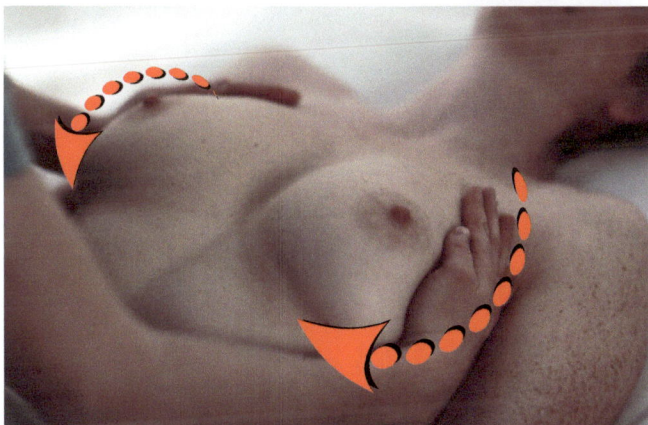

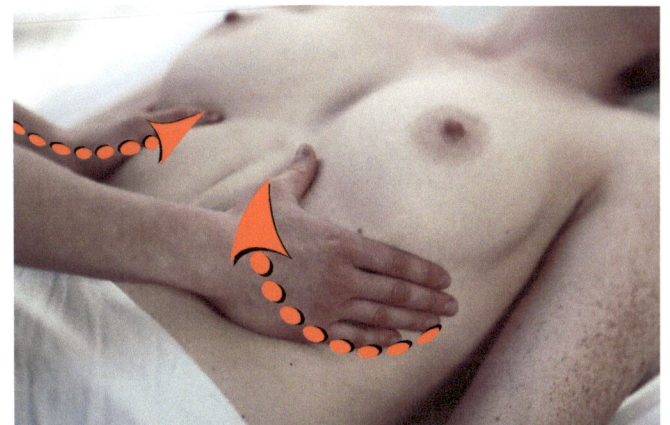

Thoracic Outlet Syndrome

What is it?

Neuromuscular compression of the Brachial Plexus, Subclavian Artery and/or Subclavian Vein, due to hypertension of Pectoralis Minor, Middle, and Anterior Scalenes. Impingement can also include the costoclavicular junction between Clavicle and first rib, posterior triangle, and Pectoralis Minor tendon.

Purpose

Decrease impingement of compression of the Brachial Plexus, Subclavian Artery and/or Subclavian Vein.

Related Pathologies

Cervical Rib Syndrome, Scalenus Anticus Syndrome, Costoclavicular Syndrome, Arterial Thoracic Outlet Syndrome, Neurogenic Thoracic Outlet Syndrome.

Indications

Neck, shoulder and arm pain, numbness and tingling of the fingers, impaired circulation to the extremities causing discoloration and impaired healing time, weakness in shoulder, arm and hand.

Endangerments

Brachial Plexus, Subclavian Artery and Internal Jugular Vein, Carotid Sinus.

Expected Outcomes

Decrease myalgia of associated structures, increase blood supply, nerve function and muscular strength.

Thoracic Outlet Treatment Options

- TX Nerve impingement: massage therapy, physical therapy, injections, Thoracic Outlet decompression surgery (1st rib resection), medication

- TX Artery impingement: massage therapy, arterial bypass and thoracic outlet decompression surgery

- TX Vein impingement: massage therapy, vein reconstruction: angioplasty, patch angioplasty, or venous bypass; thoracic outlet decompression surgery

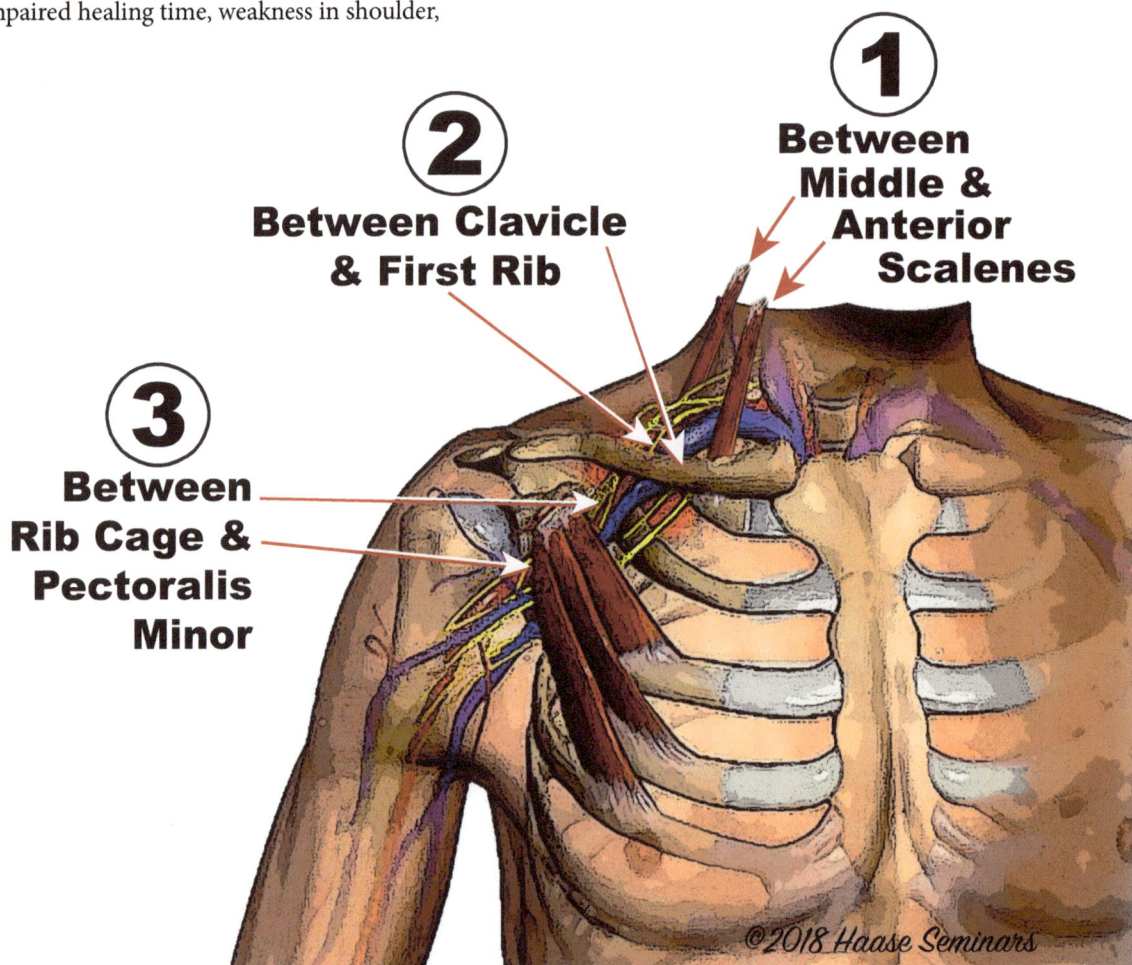

1 Between Middle & Anterior Scalenes

2 Between Clavicle & First Rib

3 Between Rib Cage & Pectoralis Minor

©2018 Haase Seminars

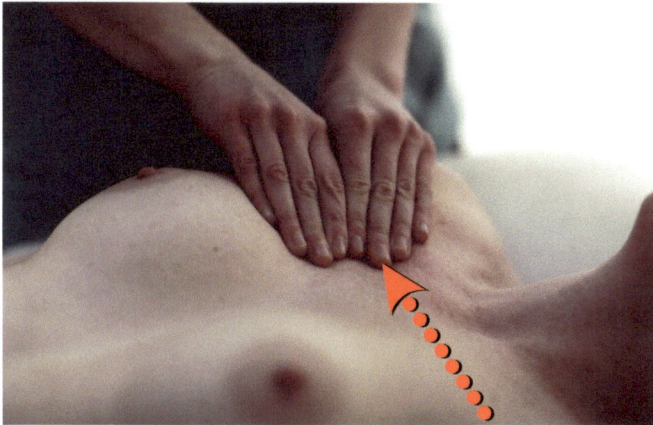

Standing adjacent to your client, scoop up the Pectoralis Major by placing your adjacent thumbs into the Axilla on the backside of the muscle.

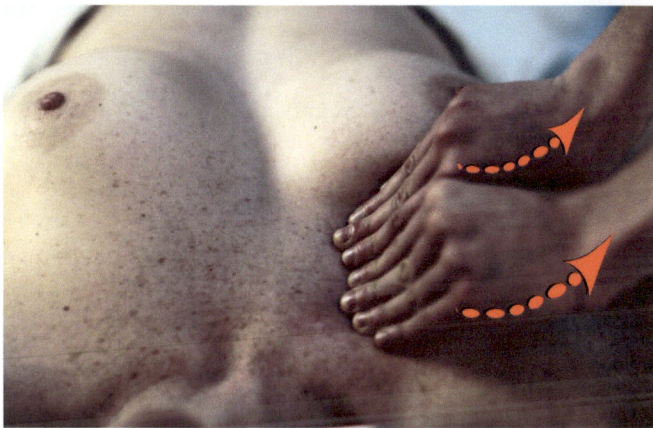

In an effort to "unroll" the Pectoralis Major, use your flat fingers on top and thumbs on the underside to grasp and lift up the Pectoralis Major, tugging gently towards yourself with myofascial intent and hold. Patiently.

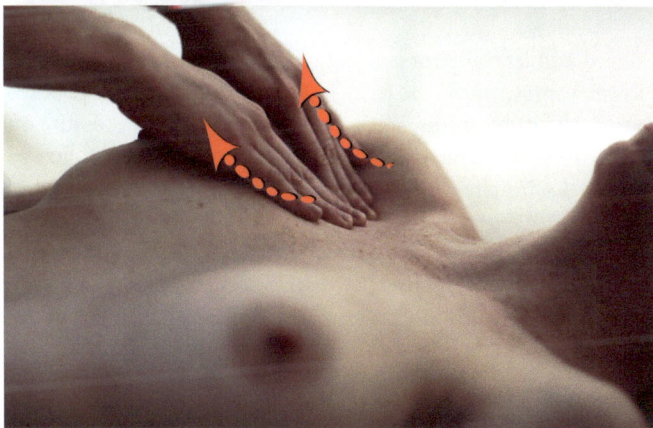

Using your flat fingers, press down firmly, just below the Clavicle, and pull down slowly as you stretch the muscle downward and away from its clavicular attachment.

With fingertips which are firmly placed together in a straight line, work the Pectoralis Major tissues which may be tight with spasm. Work the same way along the Sternum as well.

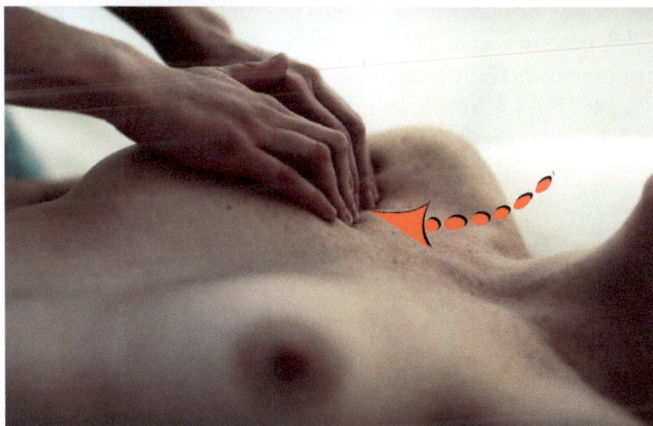

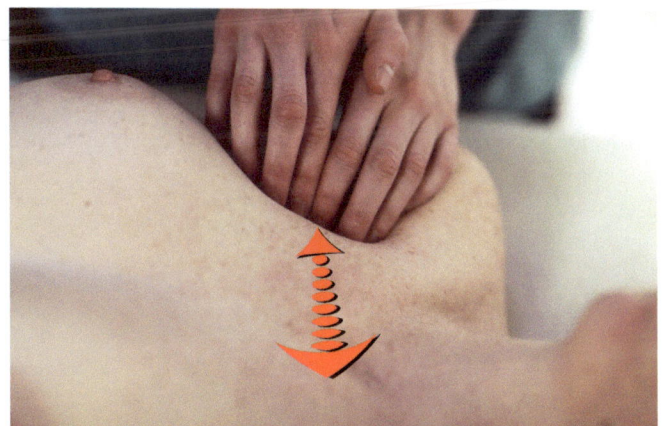

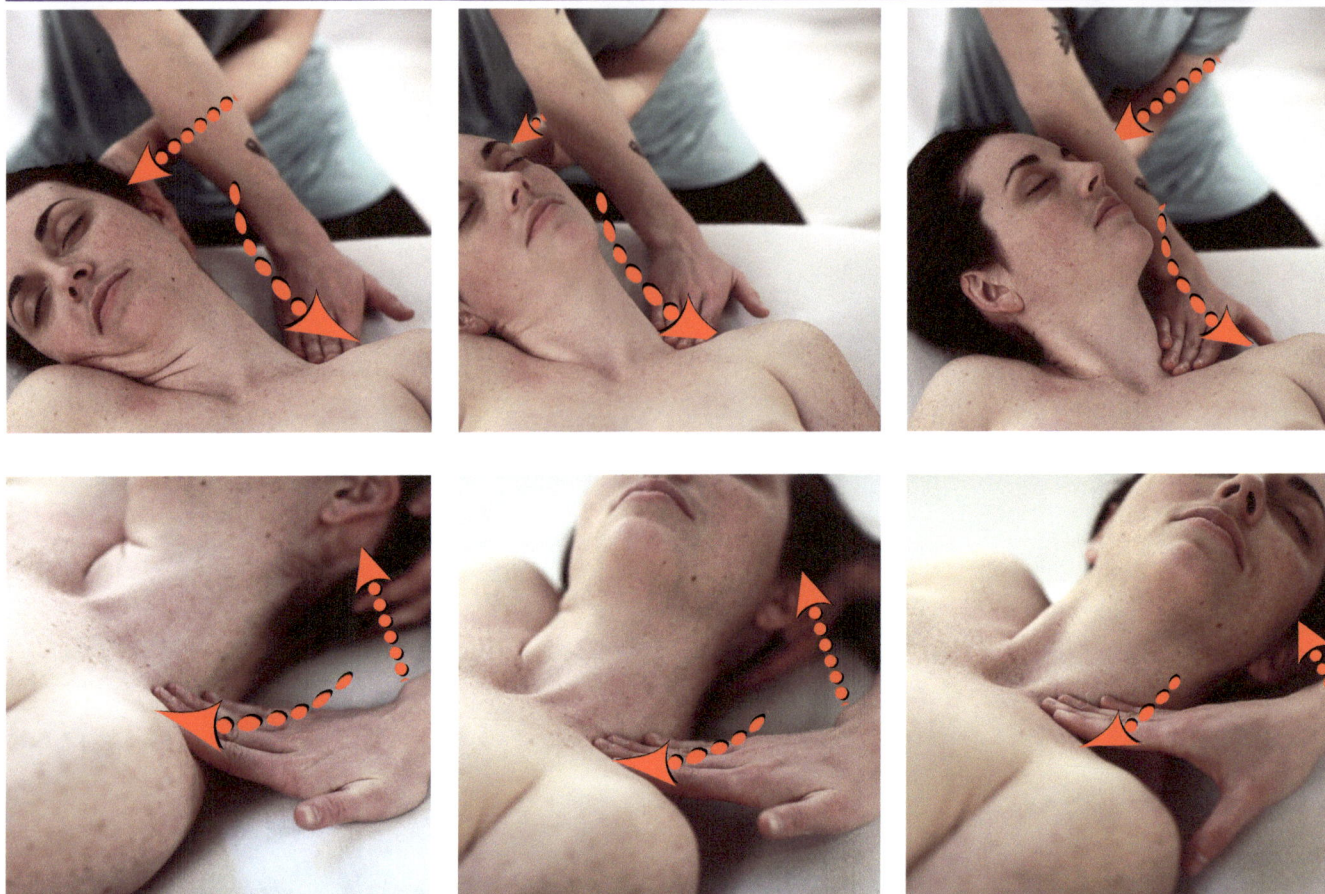

To specifically evaluate and treat the Scalenes, sit at the head of the table with your client lying supine. Place your client's head in your left hand, resting on the table, as they place their left hand under their bottom to ensure the shoulder stays in place.

As they continue to look toward the ceiling, gradually bring their right ear toward their right shoulder (right lateral flexion of the cervical spine). Once you reach the end-feel, roll their head the rest of the way to the right. The muscles on the left side of the lateral neck should show signs of tension.

With the flat finger bones of your right hand pointing towards the ceiling (in a "stop" gesture) apply pressure on the posterior aspect of the soft lateral area known as the "Posterior Triangle", outlined by the Trapezius, SCM and Clavicle.

Posterior Scalene: (above left) As your client's head is laterally flexed and laterally rotated to the right, press your flat-fingers inward and towards the left while you press the head/neck towards the right. If this causes discomfort, back the pressure off and rub with gentle cross-fiber friction movements followed by gentle stretches.

Middle Scalene: (above center) As you continue to cradle your client's head in your left hand, position the head so the client's nose is pointing toward the ceiling, then take up the slack. Again, you will use the length of your fingers to press in and towards the left as you press the head toward the right.

Anterior Scalene: (above right) Continue cradling your client's head in your left hand with the neck laterally flexed to the right and carefully position the head to look towards the left. Repeat the pressure into the scalenes and towards the right while you press their head towards the right.

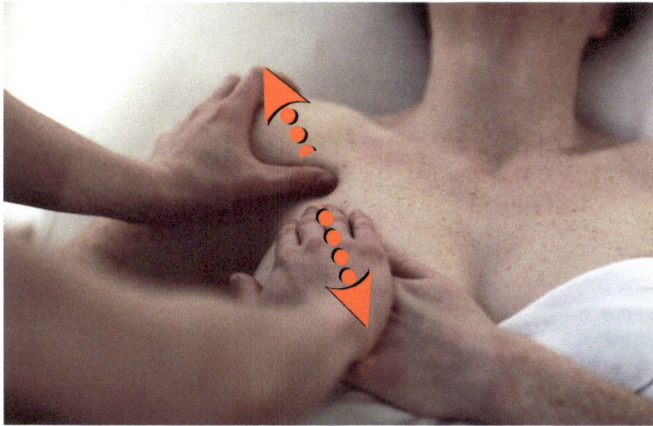

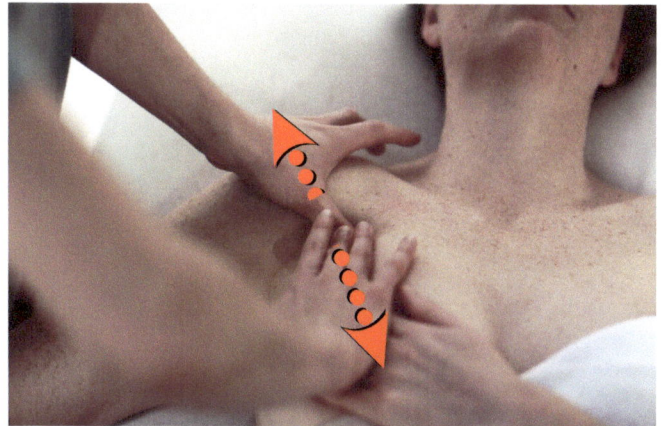

To lengthen Pectoralis Minor's fascial sheath, stand to your client's right hand side along the side of the table. Have your client place their left hand over their right breast and ensure they keep their fingers and thumb snugly together, creating a "work surface" for you to rest the heel of your right hand.

As you use the fingertips of your right hand to draw the tissue towards itself, use your left thumb to stretch the upper fibers of

the muscle in the opposite direction. (Superiorly)

Next, as you keep your right hand in place, press into any spasms and trigger points, using the fingers of your left hand for reinforcement. Work along the entire muscle belly, pressing each point for 3-6 seconds before moving along to the next.

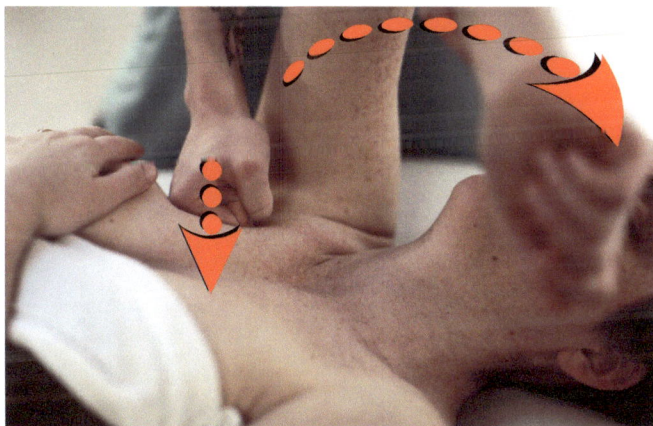

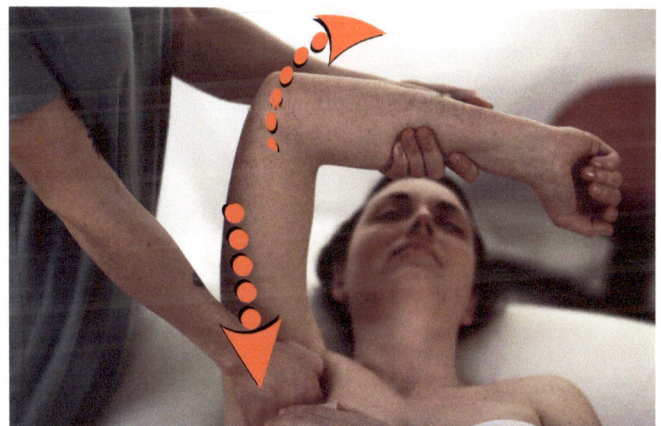

With your client's hand still covering their right breast, lift their right upper arm into a vertical position with their forearm hovering horizontally as you grasp it securely with your left hand close to their elbow.

To ensure your Pectoralis Minor stretch does not cause stretch

marks, use your right hand to make a "hard fist". Gently place it with gentle pressure on the skin over the lower portion of the Pectoralis Minor. Gently drag the skin 1/2 to 1" superiorly before pressing down firmly into the muscle belly. Hold the muscle in place with your fist as you bring their right arm up and over their head, similar to a "martial arts block".

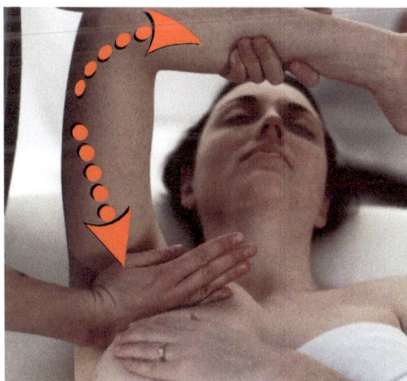

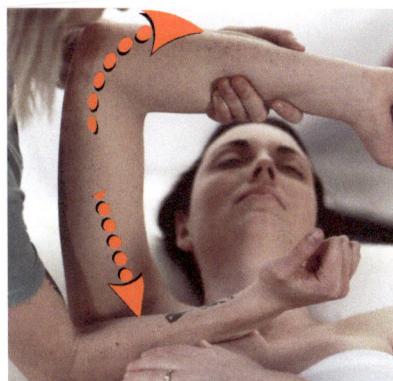

Variations of Contact

- Use the flat, smooth bone of your Ulna to press and hold the muscle (immediate left)

- Use the Pisiform bone on the edge of your hand to press down on the muscle (far left)

- Use your *hard fist* with your fingers tucked inside your palm (above)

Thoracic Outlet Breast Massage Sequence

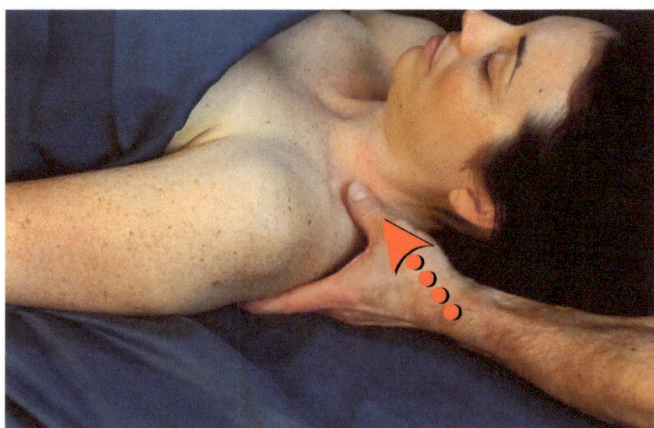

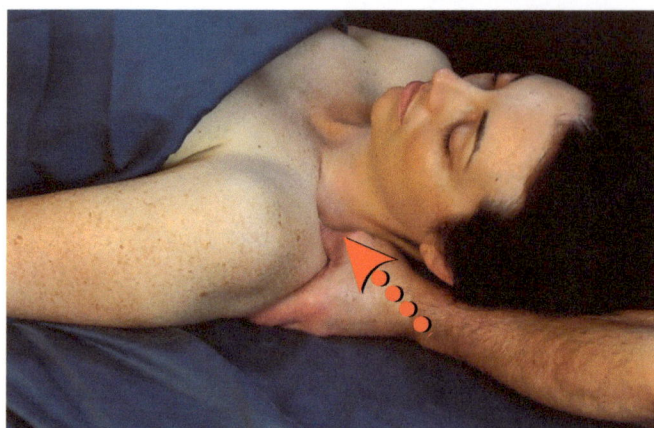

First Rib ROM: This technique is to move the first rib through its *range of motion* only. It is *not* an *adjustment* or *manipulation.*

Begin by resting your patient's head on your RIGHT hand while you slide your LEFT hand, palm up, under their LEFT shoulder until your **Locked Thumb** comes to rest in the center of the triangle.

Slide your patient's head toward your LEFT wrist as you slide your the **thumb print** of your LEFT **Locked Thumb** into the posterior triangle.

Continue pressing inward in the direction of their feet and hold for up to two minutes. Decrease the duration if your hand becomes fatigued or your patient is uncomfortable.

If you feel the bony resistance of your patient's first rib lying *just below* the skin, it likely means the rib has rotated upwards which can compress the Brachial Plexus nerve bundle.

This technique *will increase Thoracic Outlet Syndrome symptoms* during the first rib rotation. Symptoms will normalize within minutes of removing pressure on the rib.

Repeat on opposite side.

Self-Care Pectoralis Minor Stretch

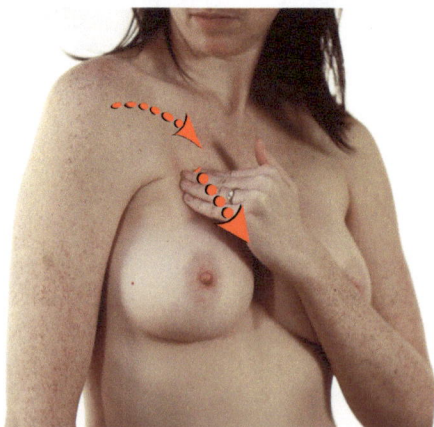

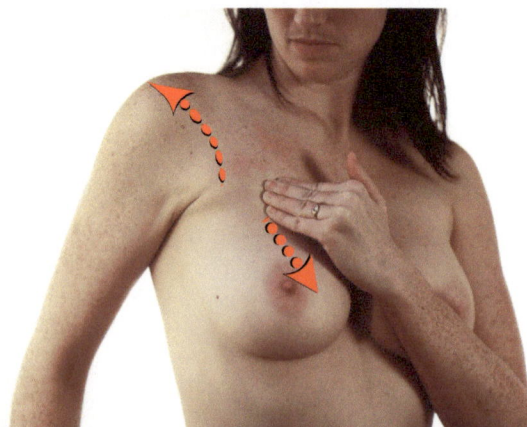

While the passive pin & stretch technique on a shortened Pectoralis Minor is quite effective, we have found clients recover at an accelerated pace if they perform self-stretching techniques.

To show your client how to perform a self-stretch on the Pectoralis Minor, first, demonstrate the location of the muscle on their *right* side so they can palpate it specifically.

Then, have your client group the fingertips of their *left* hand, keeping each of their four fingertips in alignment. Have them

then move their right shoulder forward as they press their fingertips into the Pectoralis Minor muscle belly.

They will then depress their left arm downwards and to the left, drawing the muscle into tension while they simultaneously pull their shoulder back, creating a stretch. *Repeat on opposite side.*

We have observed most clients and patients gaining the most relief by performing this stretch at a rate of approximately 3-seconds per stretch, 30-seconds per side, 3-times daily.

©2020 Haase Myotherapy® – Haase & Associates, Inc.

Working with Extreme Scar Tissue

Purpose

Increase circulation and expedite healing; reduce itchiness; reduce burn-related pain and reduce anxiety; boost body image and improve comfort levels with touch; diminish scar tissue numbness, edema, and dysfunction of compensatory structures (related to/resulting from the injury)

Related Pathologies

Depression, increased susceptibility to infection, sepsis, necrotic nerves, muscles, and blood vessels

Indications

Maturation phase of healing

Endangerments

Skin tearing and bacterial infection

Expected Outcome

Reduce fibroblast activity and decrease scar vascularity; assist collagen remodel with collagen synthesis and breakdown balancing; improve function of affected muscle, nerves, and blood vessels

---

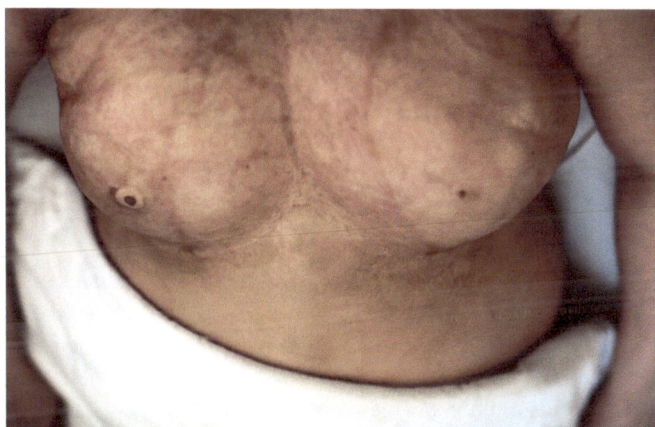

When working with visible burn-type scar tissue, the technique is the easy part, but "patience is a virtue". Regardless of whether the scars are resulting from fire or from radiation treatment, the treatment is virtually the same.

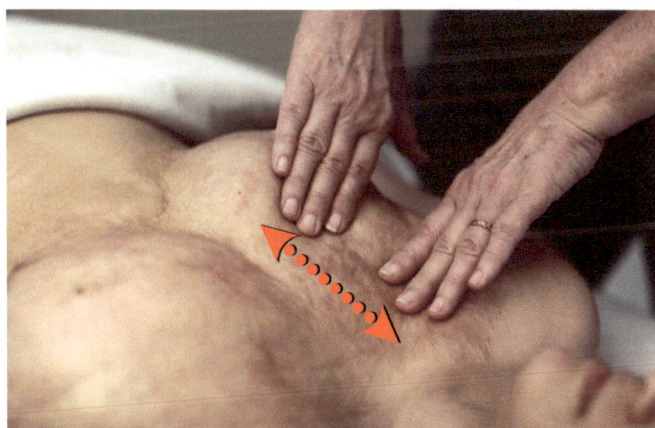

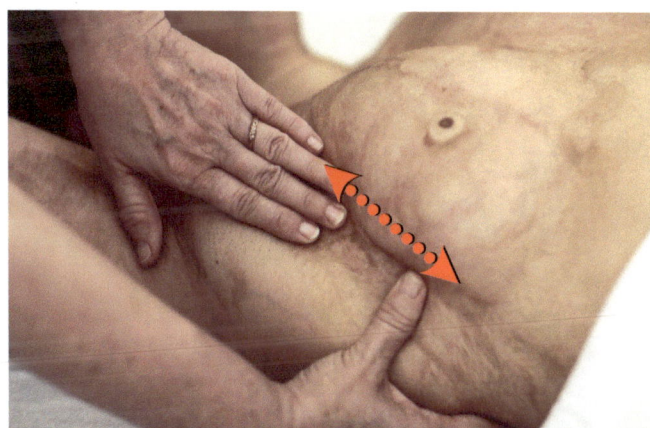

Notes

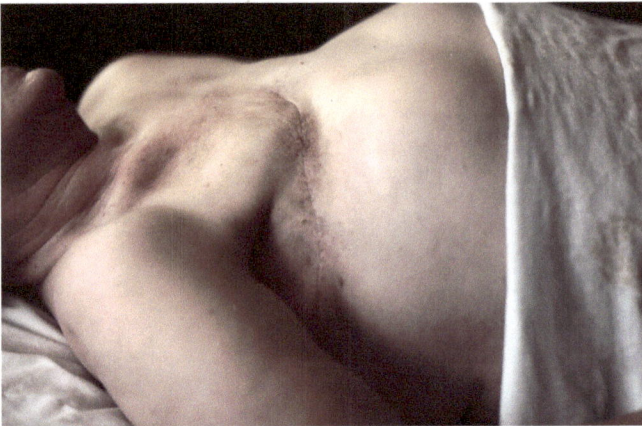

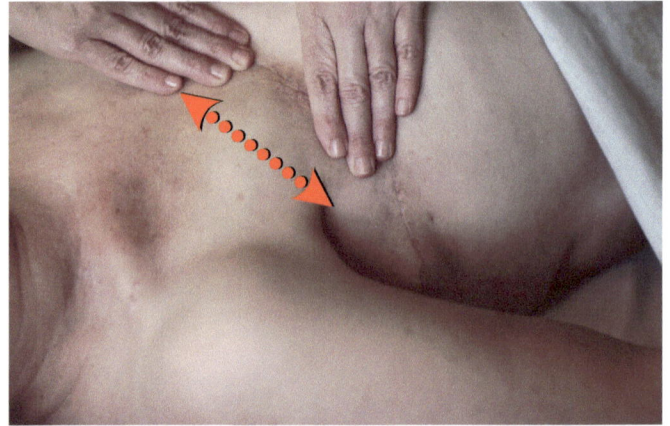

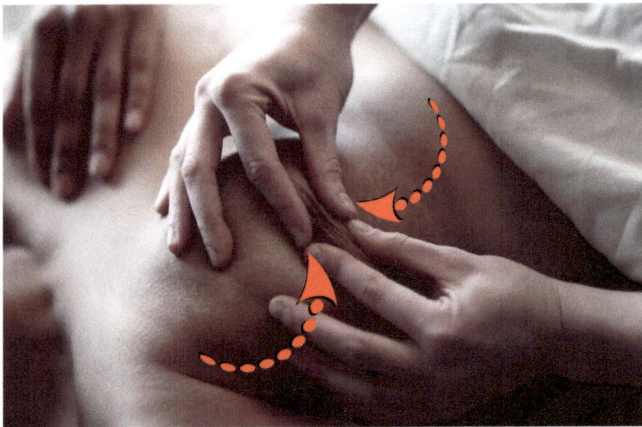

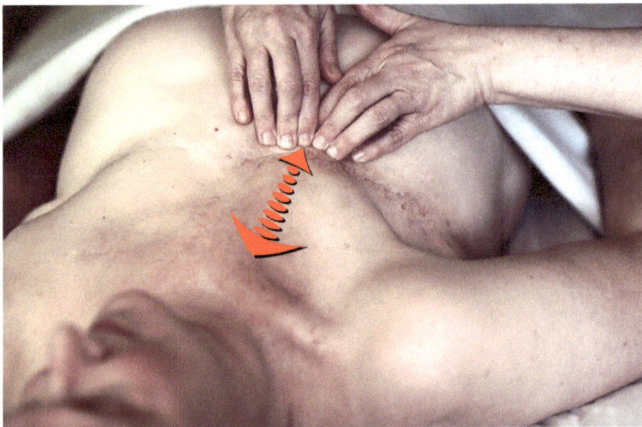

Scar Tissue Treatment Considerations

Work your client's tissue with combinations of technique appropriate for the type of scar tissue, current scar tissue condition, your client's current state of health, concurrent health diagnosis' and/or treatments, and current medications.

Treating Post Cancer Treatment Scars

Radiation Burns

Wait to treat tissue which has been burned by radiation for 6-8 weeks or until the doctor is comfortable with your client receiving massage. Approach the tissue as though it had been burned by actual fire. It would be wise to ensure radiation treatments did not decrease bone density. If density has been compromised, bone breakage is a possibility given enough force.

Chemotherapy

Chemotherapy weakens the tissues and structures of the body as much as 5-years or longer after treatment concludes. If your client asks for deep work and is currently receiving chemotherapy or has recently completed treatment, err on the side of caution when it comes to satiating your client's need for deep work.

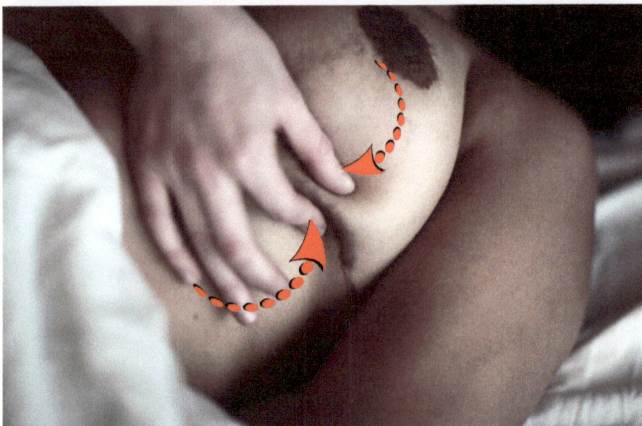

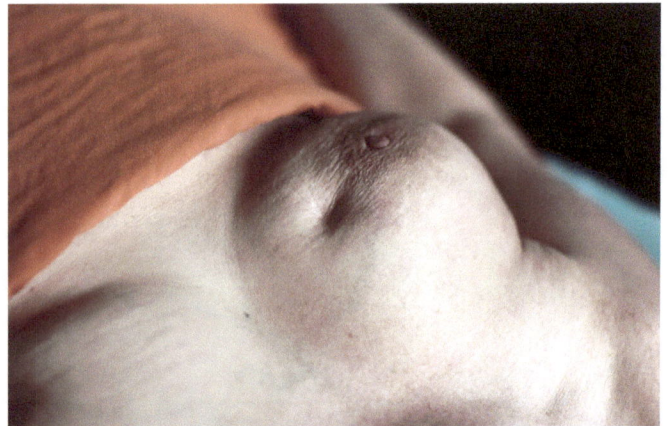

Scar Tissue Techniques

- Cross-Fiber Friction
- Pin & Stretch (local)
- Knuckle-Knurling ("Graston-like" with knuckles)
- Deep Fascial Glide w/Fingertips
- Fascial Tug
- Skin Rolling
- Pinch & Tug

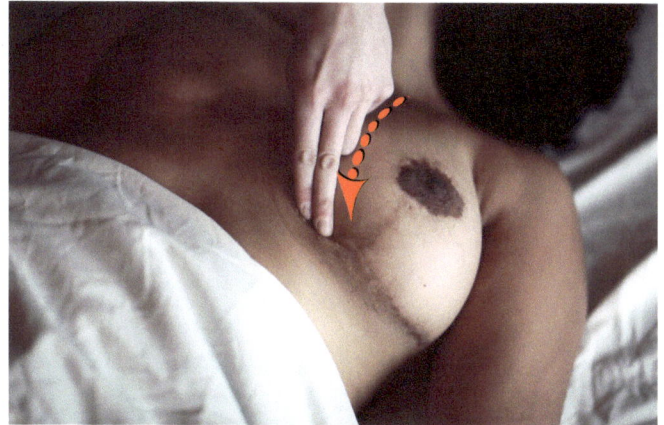

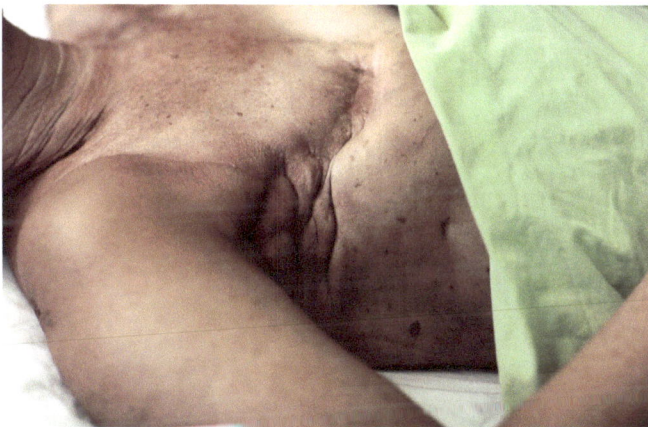

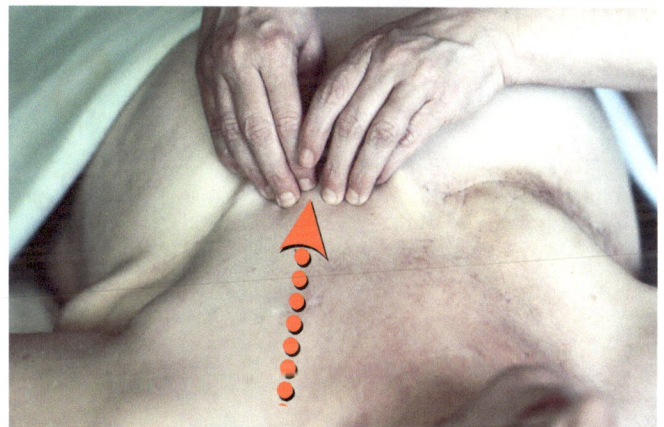

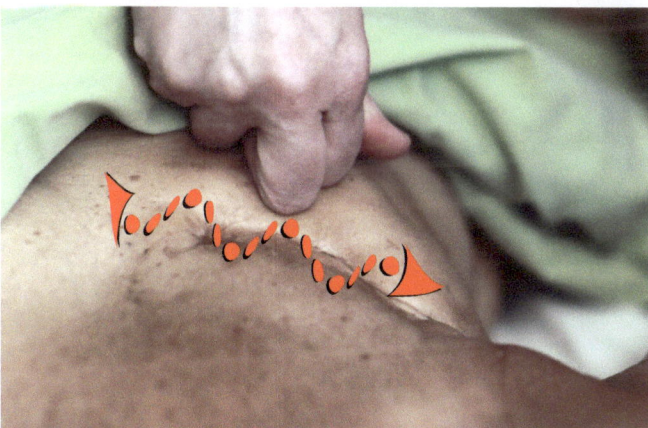

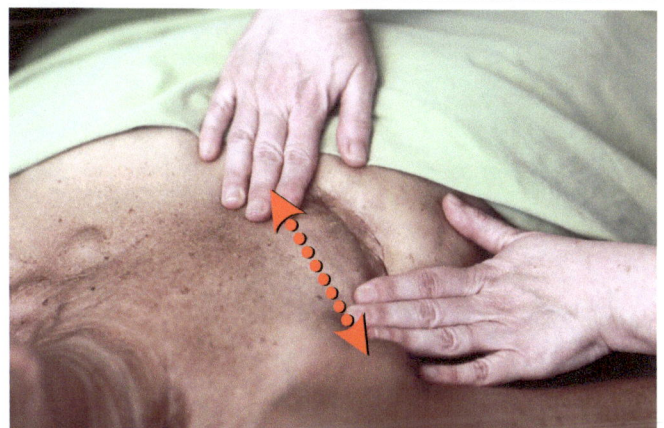

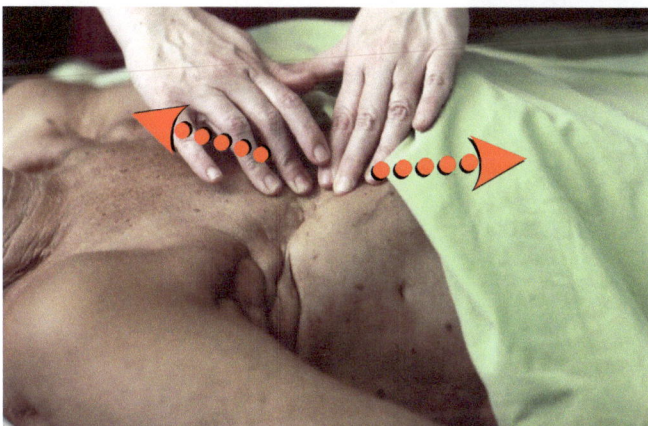

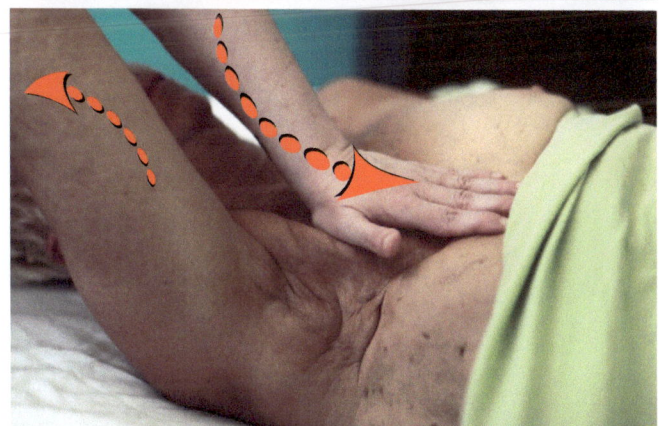

Treatment Frequency

The self-massage treatment sequence should be taught to the client as the therapist guides the client through each of the steps, ensuring correct positions and pressure. Although the same techniques can be actively applied by the therapist, the client will receive maximum benefit in the treatment of capsular contracture when they perform the self-massage sequence daily.

Purpose

Prevent and diminish scar tissue, capsule formation around implant; stimulate lymph flow and drainage; provide post-op and preventative care; myalgia; and afford an opportunity for routine breast health with self-examination.

Related Pathologies

Cancers; breast trauma; radiation; post-surgical complications like hematoma (broken blood vessels under the skin), seroma (collection of fluid under the skin), and bacterial infection; autoimmune disorders like lupus; inadequate skin coverage or using too large an implant for the amount of skin coverage; and silicone molecules that leach into the pocket holding the implant (primarily an issue with older silicone gel implants).

Indications

High-rising implant; increasing firmness; tight or painful breast sensation; round, almost "ball-like" implant appearance; and visible ripping, burning, or pain.

Endangerments

Rupture of implant and damage to surrounding glandular tissues: Caution should be given to avoid damage to lymph nodes, vessels and glandular structure. Caution when working with thin skin due to cancer treatments.

Expected Outcome

Decrease scar tissue, myalgia, and other symptoms; inhibit contracture, preventing the condition from worsening.

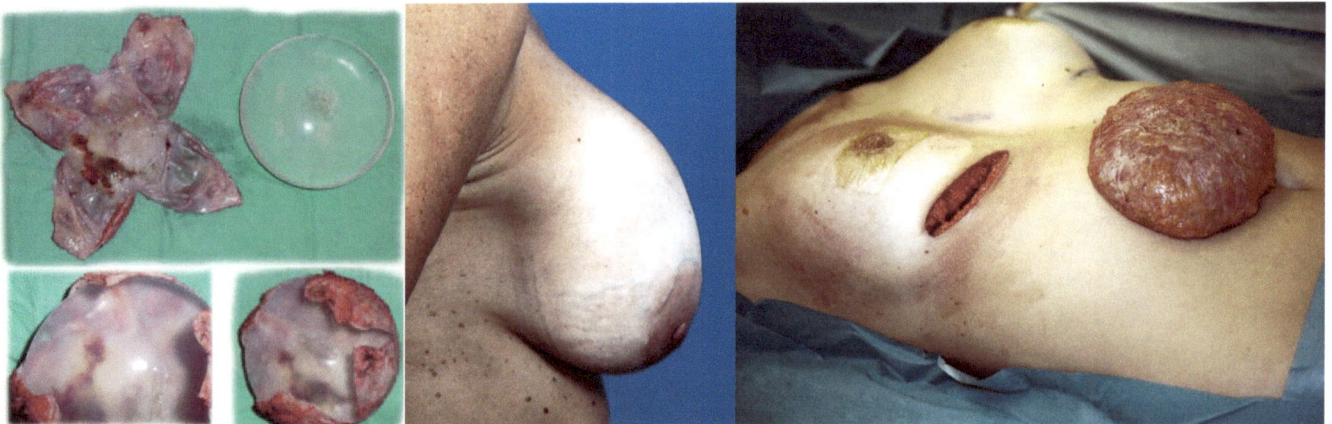

Notes

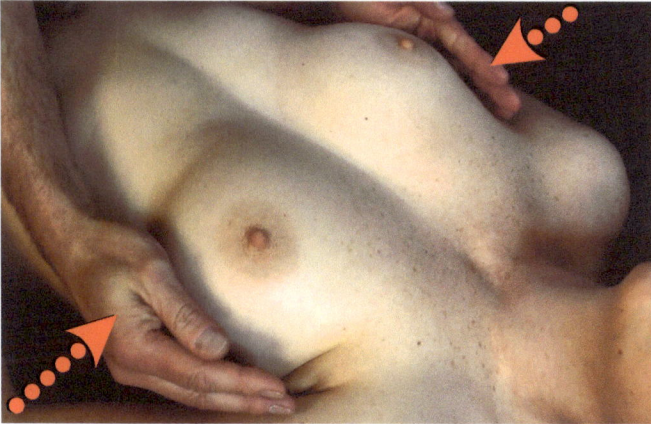

Standing table-side, press your hands on the lateral sides of the breasts, fingers pointing superiorly. Press the breasts together

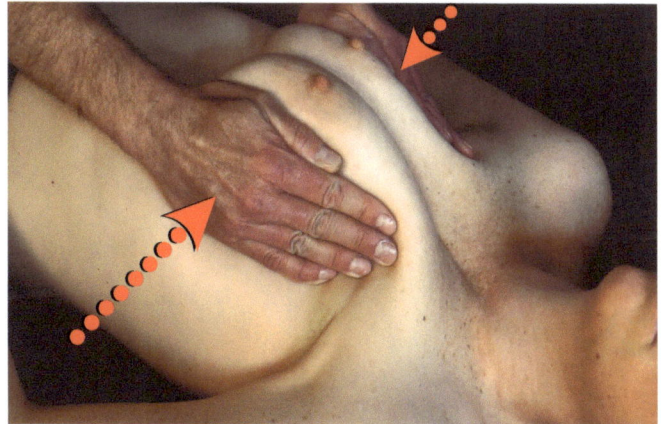

for 3-seconds with firm pressure, release and repeat for a total of 30-seconds.

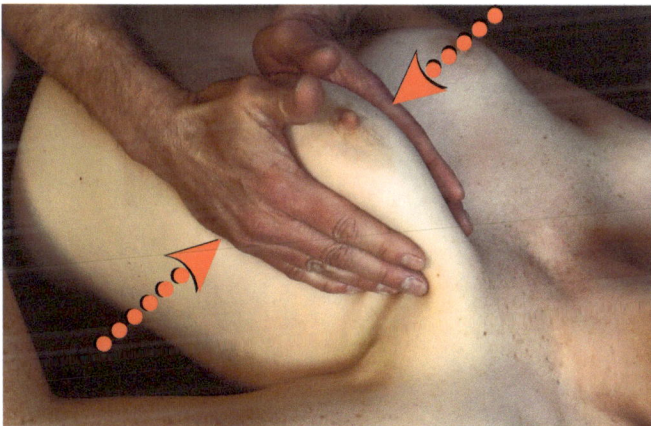

Repeat the double-breast press on each breast separately with the same amount of pressure as above.

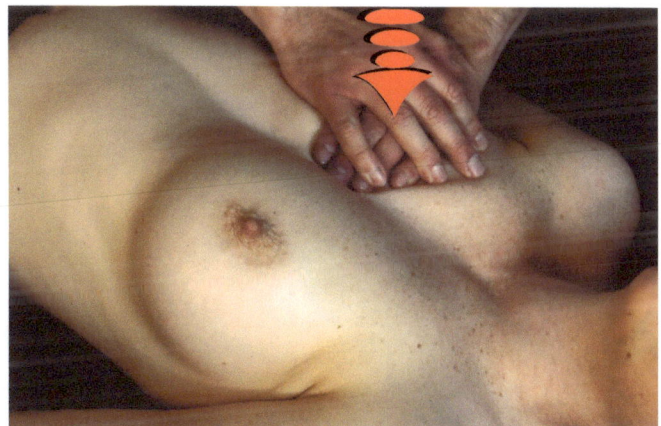

Use both hands to press one breast for a 3-second hold, repeating for a total of 30-seconds on one side, then repeat on the opposite side.

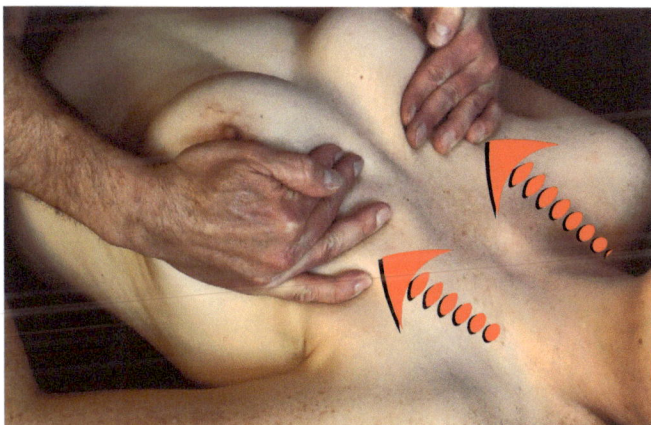

Standing table-side facing your client's head, place your cupped hands at the top of the breasts, just above the breast implants. Pull the breasts down inferiorly, away from their head and in the direction of their feet, with firm pressure. Hold for 3-seconds and repeat for a total of 30-seconds.

Notes

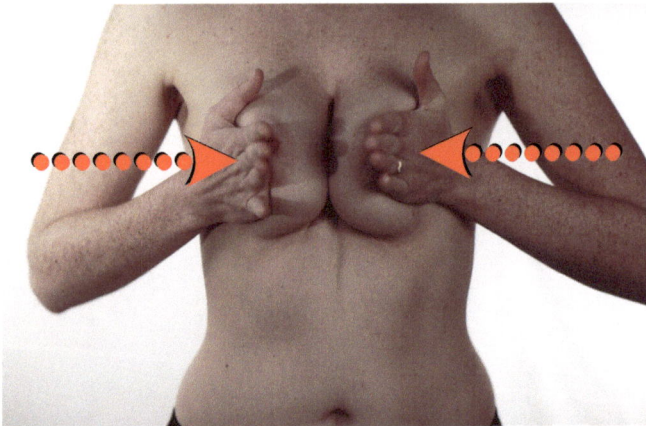

Press your hands on the outsides of your breasts, fingers pointing forward. Press the breasts together for 3-seconds, release and repeat for 30-seconds.

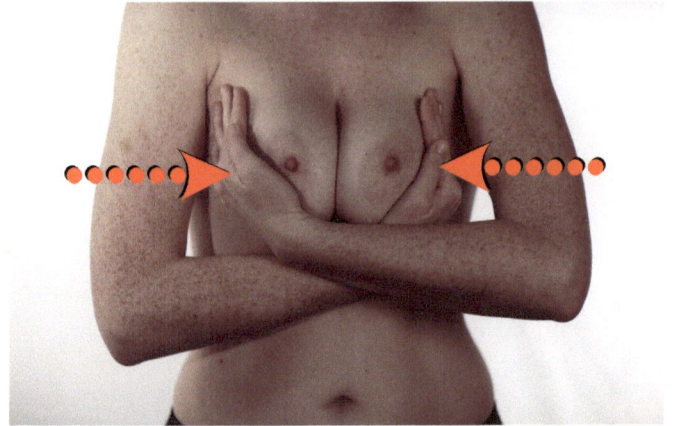

With crossed arms, use your hands to cup the outside (lateral aspect) of your breasts, press them together for 3-seconds, release and repeat for 30-seconds.

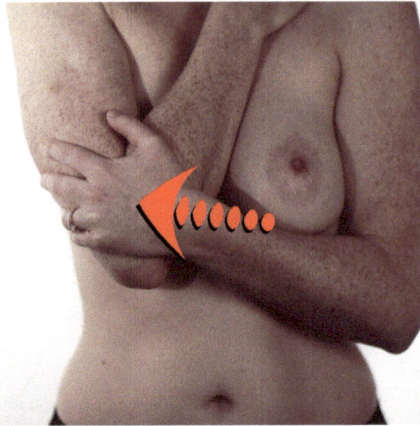

Place your right hand on your left shoulder. Use your left hand to press your right elbow into your breast and hold for 3-seconds. Repeat for 30-seconds. Repeat on the opposite side.

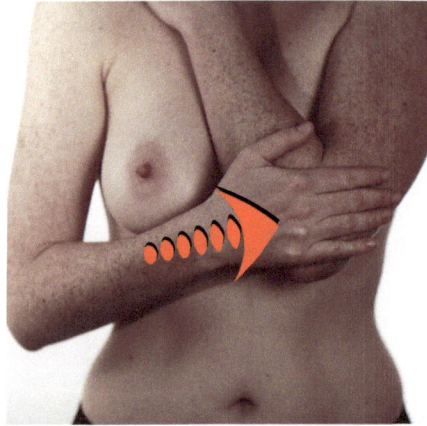

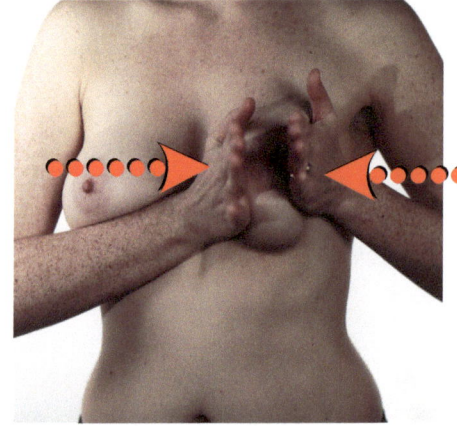

Similarly to the first step, use both hands to press one breast for a 3-second hold repeating for 30-seconds. Repeat on the opposite side.

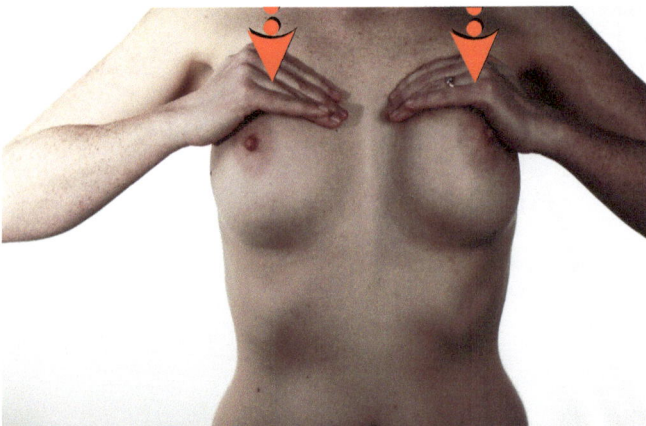

Place your cupped hands at the top of your breasts, just above your breast implants.

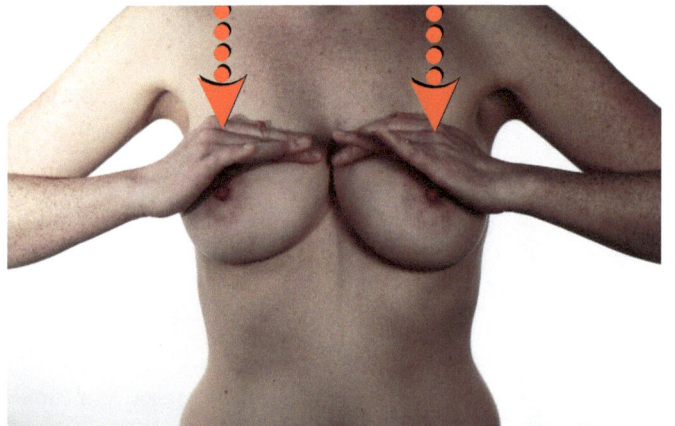

Press downward firmly, holding for 3-seconds and repeat for 30-seconds.

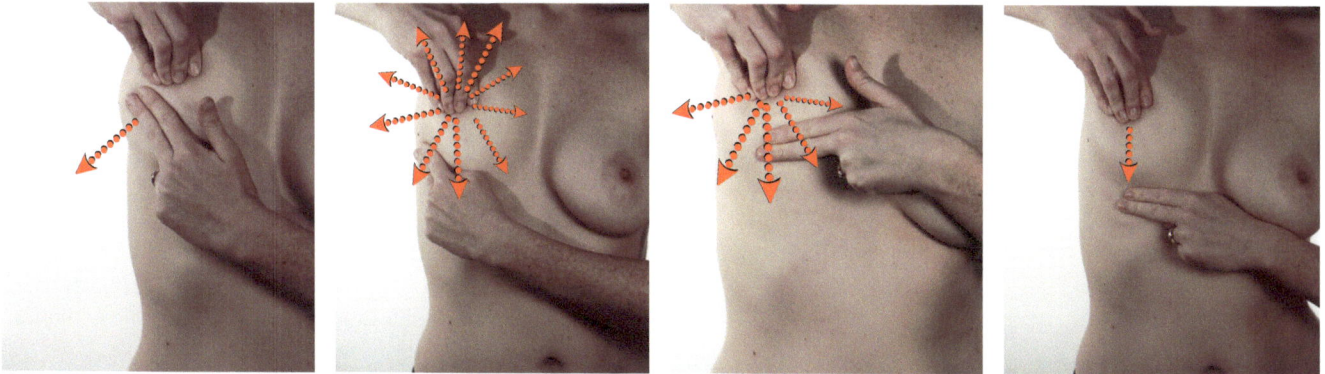

Step One: Use your fingers to gently smooth away from the nipple, using no more pressure than what you would apply to your eyelid.

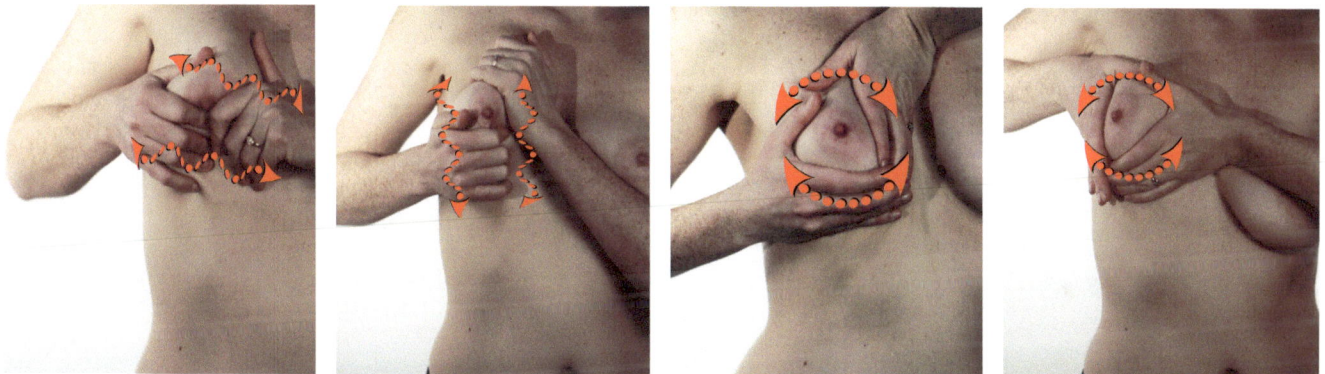

Step Two: Gently massage the breast with a kneading motion, using lifting and pressing movements.

Step Three: Slowly and carefully use your hands to gently twist the breast in a clock-wise and counterclockwise direction.

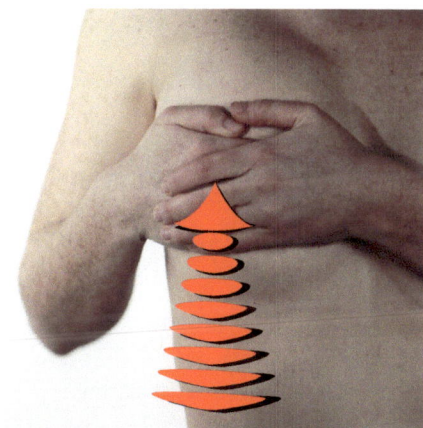

Step Four: Use both hands as shown to apply several, moderate pressure, compressions.

Notes

Section Three: Sequence Reviews

Essential Breast Massage Sequence

1. To begin stimulating lymph flow in the upper chest and breast areas, standing adjacent to your client facing towards their head. Place one hand on the Sternum with fingers firmly close together pointing toward your client's head.

2. Tap rhythmically with your fingers against the back of your hand, transferring the percussive movement into your client's Sternum, stimulating lymph flow.

3. Gently place overlapped hands on top of Sternum with full palmar contact, placing one hand directly over the other.

4. Gently press downward. Slowly press and release at a rate of about one compression every second, creating a smooth pumping action.

5. Continue with the same pumping compressions as you work around the breast and Pectoralis Major, working from the opposite side of which you are standing. Be sure to work up to and just under the clavicle with your direction moving up the Sternum, then laterally over the upper chest.

6. Using one hand to stabilize the breast, use two fingers on your other hand to gently squeegee the superficial tissues of the breast, gliding directly away from the nipple. Work all the way around the breast.

7. With both hands, begin massaging the entire breast with petrissage strokes, being sure to gently mobilize the tissue.

8. In an effort to benefit the Cooper's Ligaments of the breast, take both hands and twist the breast into gentle traction. Twist both clockwise and counterclockwise in alternate directions, holding each twist a 1-2 seconds before redirecting the twist in the other direction.

9. With both hands, use compressions, each lasting 1-2 seconds, pressing downward into your client's chest until the breast appears nearly flat.

10. Depending on your preference, you can either press with your hands encircling the Areola*, or with your hands completely covering the Areola. The preferred method is to include the Areola with each compression.

11. Finish the sequence with a traditional Hawaiian Lomi-Lomi smoothing effleurage stroke from the head of the table. Begin with your flat hands pressing down on the upper chest, gliding down the Sternum, down and over the lower abdomen.

12. With hands mirroring each other on both sides of the anterior torso, glide laterally over the External Obliques and back up along Serratus Anterior.

13. Continue the stroke along the lateral breasts, gathering together at the Sternum, just below the Menubrial Notch, and over the Deltoids, finishing along the lateral neck muscles, giving them a gentle squeeze.

14. Similarly, you will repeat the previous Hawaiian Lomi-Lomi effleurage stroke from the side of the table, as you stand with your backside towards the client's feet.

15. With your flat hands, side by side, begin at the center of the Sternum, gliding superiorly, up and then laterally over and around the breasts.

16. The stroke finishes as your hands come together, gathering together at the lower ribcage.

Thoracic Outlet Massage Sequence

Pectoralis Major

1. Standing adjacent to your client, scoop up the Pectoralis Major by placing your adjacent thumbs into the Axilla on the backside of the muscle.

2. In an effort to "unroll" the Pectoralis Major, use your flat fingers on top and thumbs on the underside to grasp and lift up the Pectoralis Major, tugging gently towards yourself with myofascial intent and hold. Patiently.

3. Using your flat fingers, press down firmly, just below the clavicle, and pull down slowly as you stretch the muscle downward and away from its Clavicular attachment.

4. With fingertips which are firmly placed together in a straight line, work the Pectoralis Major tissues which may be tight with spasm. Work the same way along the Sternum as well.

5. Repeat on other side.

Scalenes

1. To specifically evaluate and treat the Scalenes, sit at the head of the table with your client lying supine. Place your client's head in your left hand, resting on the table, as they place their left hand under their bottom to ensure the shoulder stays in place. As they continue to look toward the ceiling, gradually bring their right ear toward their right shoulder (right lateral flexion of the cervical spine). Once you reach the end-feel, roll their head the rest of the way to the right. The muscles on their lateral neck should show signs of tension.

2. With the flat finger bones of your right hand pointing towards the ceiling (in a "stop" gesture) apply pressure on the posterior aspect of the soft lateral area known as the "Posterior Triangle", outlined by the Trapezius, SCM, and Clavicle.

3. Posterior Scalene: As your client's head is laterally flexed and laterally rotated to the right, press your flat-fingers inward and towards the left while you press the head/neck towards the right. If this causes discomfort, back the pressure off and rub with gentle cross-fiber friction movements followed by gentle stretches.

4. Middle Scalene: As you continue to cradle your client's head in your left hand, position the head so their nose is pointing toward the ceiling, then take up the slack. Again, you will use the length of your fingers to press in and towards the left as you press the head toward the right.

5. Anterior Scalene: Continue cradling your client's head in your left hand with the neck laterally flexed to the right and carefully position the head to look towards the left. Repeat the pressure into the Scalenes and towards the right while you press their head towards the right.

6. Repeat on other side.

Pectoralis Minor

1. To lengthen Pectoralis Minor fascial sheath, stand to your client's right-hand side along the side of the table. Have your client place their left hand over their right breast and ensure they keeps their fingers and thumb snugly together, creating a "work surface" for you to rest the heel of your right hand.

2. As you use the fingertips of your right hand to draw the tissue towards itself, use your left thumb to stretch the upper fibers of the muscle in the opposite direction. (Superiorly)

3. Next, as you keep your right hand in place, press into any spasms and trigger points, using the fingers of your left hand for reinforcement. Work along the entire muscle belly, pressing each point for 3-6 seconds before moving along to the next.

4. With your client's hand still covering their right breast, lift their right upper arm into a vertical position with their forearm hovering horizontally as you grasp it securely with your left hand close to their elbow.

5. To ensure your Pectoralis Minor stretch does not cause stretch marks, use your right hand to make a "hard fist". Gently place it with gentle pressure on the skin over the lower portion of the Pectoralis Minor. Gently drag the skin 1/2 to 1" superiorly before pressing down firmly into the muscle belly. Hold the muscle in place with your fist as you bring their right arm up and over their head, similar to a "martial arts block".

6. Remember your options for applying pressure on the muscle belly:

   ► Use the flat, smooth bone of your Ulna to press and hold the muscle.

   ► Use the Pisiform bone on the edge of your hand to press down on the muscle.

   ► Use using your *hard fist* with your fingers tucked inside your palm.

7. Repeat on other side.

Working with Extreme Scar Tissue

Scar Tissue Techniques:

► Cross-Fiber Friction

► Pin & Stretch (local)

► Knuckle-Knurling ("Graston-like" knuckles)

► Deep Fascial Glide with Fingertips

► Fascial Tug

► Skin Rolling

► Pinch & Tug

Capsular Contracture Self-Massage

1. Press your hands on the outsides of your breasts, fingers pointing forward. Press the breasts together for 3-seconds, release and repeat for 30-seconds.

2. With crossed arms, use your hands to cup the outside (lateral aspect) of your breasts, press them together for 3-seconds, release and repeat for 30-seconds.

3. Place your right hand on your left shoulder. Use your left hand to press your right elbow into your breast and hold for 3-seconds. Repeat for 30-seconds. Repeat on the opposite side.

4. Similarly to the first step, use both hands to press one breast for a 3-second hold repeating for 30-seconds. Repeat on the opposite side.

5. Place your cupped hands at the top of your breasts, just above your breast implants.

6. Press downward firmly, holding for 3-seconds and repeat for 30-seconds.

Capsular Contracture Massage

1. Standing table-side, press your hands on the lateral sides of the breasts, fingers pointing superior. Press the breasts together for 3-seconds with firm pressure, release and repeat for a total of 30-seconds.

2. Repeat the double-breast press on each breast separately with the same amount of pressure as above.

3. Use both hands to press one breast for a 3-second hold, repeating for a total of 30-seconds on one side, then repeat on the opposite side.

4. Standing table-side facing your client's head, place your cupped hands at the top of the breasts, just above the breast implants. Pull the breasts down inferiorly, away from their head and in the direction of their feet, with firm pressure. Hold for 3-seconds and repeat for a total of 30-seconds.

Essential Breast Health Self-Massage

1. Use your fingers to gently smooth away from the nipple, using no more pressure than what you would apply to your eyelid.

2. Gently massage the breast with a kneading-like motion, using lifting and pressing movements.

3. Slowly and carefully use your hands to gently twist the breast in a clock-wise and counterclockwise direction.

4. Use overlapped hands to apply several, moderate pressure, compressions to move out more pressure fluids.

Notes

Essential Breast Massage Sequence

- Hand on Sternum, finger tap
- 1-second rhythmic pump hand on hand
- Continue UP Sternum and around upper pecs
- 2-finger squeegee
- Petrissage entire breast
- Alternating twist
- Breast compression
- Encircle Areola
- Complete
- Lomi-Lomi Effleurage from head of table
- Down Sternum
- Over abdomen
- Up sides
- Gather at Sternum
- Over shoulder
- Posterior neck
- Lomi-Lomi Effleurage from SIDE of table
- Start at Sternum
- Up around breasts
- Gather at upper abdomen

Thoracic Outlet Massage Sequence

- Unfurling Pectoralis Major
- Inferior Clavicle *fingerprint* tug
- Fingertip drag Pectoralis Major
- Scalene Sequence
- Pin & Stretch LOCAL Pectoralis Minor
- TP w/fingertip along Pectoralis Minor
- Pin & Stretch Pectoralis Minor w/arm block
  - ▶ Fist
  - ▶ Pisiform bone
  - ▶ Forearm

Self-Massage:
Teach Client Pectoralis Minor Stretch

- Align fingertips
- Shoulder forward
- Palpate muscle
- Press in and downward
- Pull SHOULDER ONLY backward

Scar Tissue

- Cross-Fiber Friction
- Pin & Stretch (local)
- Knuckle-Knurling ("Graston-like" with knuckles)
- Deep Fascial Glide w/Fingertips
- Fascial Tug
- Skin Rolling
- Pinch & Tug

Capsular Contracture Massage

- Press your hands on lateral sides of both breasts, fingers pointing superior.
  - ▶ Press the breasts together for 3-seconds, release and repeat for a total of 30-seconds.
- Press your hands on the sides of *one breast*, fingers pointing superior for 3-seconds, release and repeat for a total of 30-seconds.
  - ▶ Repeat on opposite breast.
- Two-handed press on one breast for a 3-second hold, repeating for a total of 30-seconds.
  - ▶ Repeat on the opposite side.
- Cupped hands at top of breasts. Pull breasts down inferiorly. Hold for 3-seconds and repeat for a total of 30-seconds.

Self-Massage:
Capsular Contracture Sequence

- Dual-breast side-squish w/forward fingers
- Cross-arm medial side-squish
- Vertical forearm press left/right
- Single-breast side-squish w/forward fingers
- Horizontal downward flat-palm press

Self-Massage:
Teach Essential Sequence

- 2-finger starburst squeegee
- Petrissage
- Twist
- Press

www.ingramcontent.com/pod-product-compliance
Lightning Source LLC
Chambersburg PA
CBHW041703200326

41518CB00002B/176